Mommy Can't Fix It: *Coping with Type One Diabetes*

By Rhonda W Fuselier

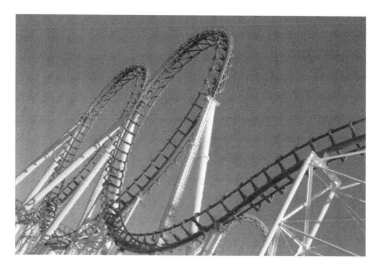

(Image courtesy of Parade.com)

This book is dedicated to my twin boys who inspire me every day. Mommy loves you, Asa and Aiden!

Special thanks to my co-pilot and husband, Jerry, for supporting me through this project. I love you more than words can express. Thanks to my friend, Melissa, for offering me constructive criticism and feedback. Thanks for being there! And, thanks to my friends in the Diabetic Community who took a few minutes of their time to give some insight into this book.

A portion of all sales of this book will go to Juvenile Diabetes Research Foundation (JDRF). Helping Make Type One Type None.

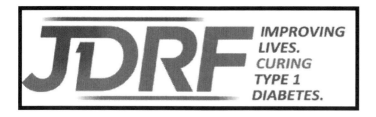

Mommy Can't Fix It:

Coping with Type One Diabetes

D-Day: One Year Later

One D-Mom's Journey

Prologue:

On February 20, 2012, my 7-year-old twin son, Aiden, was formally diagnosed with Type One Diabetes. As I begin to write this, it has been almost a year since his diagnosis. I have traveled through a wide spectrum of emotions and have waffled back and forth through Elizabeth Kubler-Ross's stages of grief (Denial, Anger, Bargaining, Depression, and Acceptance).

When a friend of mine's son was diagnosed, I watched her traverse through this complicated new world, and the idea for the book was born. I was inspired to write by living this life and reading others' books and blogs. I want to tell the tale with some experiential advice, a little background knowledge, and a lot of emotion. I want to open people's eyes to what it is like to mother a Type One Diabetic, and if this book helps even one D-Mom not feel alone or crazy for how she is feeling, then I have won!

My name is Rhonda, and this is my journey.

Chapter One: Beginning of Our Journey

Background

A little about me: I went to college immediately out of high school. Initially I was a Psychology major, but after one year, I changed my major to nursing. I graduated with a Bachelor's Degree in Nursing in 1997, Magna Cum Laude, from Texas Christian University in Fort Worth, Texas.   My specialty is Women's Services including Postpartum/Gyn, Well and Sick Newborns and Labor and Delivery. While in college, I worked as a phlebotomist in a hospital laboratory. We did ALL the blood sugar checks on all patients, so I became quite adept at finger sticks and venipunctures. I learned to recognize signs of low blood sugar, and I saw many diabetics hospitalized for diabetic complications and diabetic ketoacidosis. In nursing school, we learned about endocrine disorders, including Diabetes. Little did I know it was a foundation that would serve me well later in my life.

In 1999 at the ripe old age of 24, I met my husband, Jerry, through an online dating website. We each had been married and each had two children from those marriages, a daughter and son each. To say it was love at first sight is a bit cliché, but I can tell you, from the moment we met, we were attached. We each knew pretty quickly that we had found the one but were both a little too gun shy to admit it yet. Jerry and I married in October of 2000, 16 months after meeting.

Jerry is healthy, and the only real family medical history he had was that his biological father has Type One Diabetes. His father, Johnny, was not part of his life until 2006, and we later learned he came from a family of six boys and one girl. Johnny was diagnosed with

T1D at age 10. None of his siblings or their children has T1D. None of Johnny's aunts or uncles has Type One Diabetes. Because his father was diabetic, Jerry was closely monitored for signs of Diabetes and complains he "got his finger poked all the danged time" when he was a kid. Needless to say, he escaped his childhood with a few pricks on his finger but no disease. Although there is some Type Two Diabetes, there is no history of Type One Diabetes in my family.

After Jerry and I were married, I entered a Master's Program to earn my Master's Degree in Nursing Administration. Also, we decided to have our own baby. We were told we were crazy because we already had four kids combined, but we wanted our own little chap. We wanted a baby we did not have to share with anyone else; a baby who tied us all together as a family. And, I love babies, so there! We had to wait a year longer than we originally thought to have that baby, but in May of 2003, our first son, Jace, was born. We were very excited! I graduated in December 2003 with a dual Master's degree in Nursing Administration and Healthcare Administration.

After Jace's birth, we left our options open regarding having another baby. We thought perhaps it would be cool to have our own daughter sometime, but we were undecided. That is when the hands of fate stepped in. In March of 2004, I discovered I was pregnant again. BIG surprise! What surprised us even more was being told during that first prenatal visit that there were TWO! Shock is the only word that describes that day. Neither of us have a history of twins in our family, so this was NOWHERE on our radars. From that moment forward, I hoped and prayed to carry my babies as long as possible, and as I did with all of my pregnancies, I made the healthiest choices possible to give my babies the best foundation possible. We did not get our girl. Instead, we were so fortunate to get two more healthy little boys. In October of 2004, at almost 36 weeks gestation, twins Asa and Aiden were born one minute apart. They each spent a little time transitioning in the Neonatal Intensive Care Unit (NICU), but overall, they were healthy. The first time I saw them in the NICU, I picked them out with nobody telling me which babies were mine. They were shrunken clones of my husband. Fair, blonde, large blue eyes. He could not deny them if he tried. (It amuses me when people suggest they look like me at all! Not so much.) We went home three-and-a-half days later to a new life with seven children total, five in the house, three in diapers.

Rule Breakers

As I mentioned, Jerry and I have no known family history of twins. Trendsetters we are, I guess. Against the statistical odds, we had twins. We were told they were fraternal twins because they did not share a placenta. I had done my research and knew that identical twins, on rare occasions, could have completely separate placentas if the embryo split incredibly early, but we were assured they were fraternal. Upon their delivery, my obstetrician even noted how the boys' placentas did not even border each other. They were on separate planes of the uterus, which almost never happens. Rule Breakers.

Throughout their infancy, we had to be diligent in how we dressed the boys. There were NO differences as you may expect with fraternal twins. We had to work very hard to not mix the babies up. At one year of age, we had our boys genetically tested and discovered that they were indeed identical twins. I was right. Less than 10% of identical twins will completely separate, and my little rule breakers defied those statistics, too! I felt this was important to know for their own medical history now and in the future.

Because of Jerry's family history, Juvenile Diabetes has always been on my radar for my step-children and our children. However, I had hoped and perhaps thought that Johnny's diabetes could have been a fluke, not a trait that would resurface. Yet, I was not naïve enough to completely ignore the history. We used to tease my mother-in-law, Connie, because anytime someone pottied too much after drinking six Capri Suns, she was convinced they were diabetic....even my first two children who were not genetically related to Jerry or his father. Because Jace is so similar to Johnny, I sort of kept a closer eye on him thinking that if anyone would get this disease, it would be him. But, I was wrong.

Shortly after turning seven, my baby Aiden began showing signs of Diabetes. In February, he was diagnosed. And, so it begins. You never think will happen to you, and then it does.

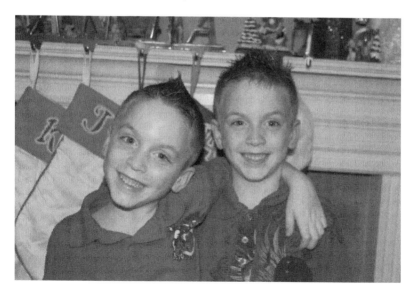

The Calm Before the Storm. Asa & Aiden, November 2011

Diagnosis Day (D-day)

As I did almost every year, in November of 2011 around Thanksgiving time, I took all my boys to the pediatrician for an annual Flu vaccination. My children have always been pretty healthy, especially my twins, but I work in a hospital and they go to public school. Germs are out there, and I want to keep them all protected. They received the Flu Mist inactivated live virus nasal vaccine. Sniff, sniff. Vaccinated. Move on.

In mid-to-late December, Aiden began this strange squinting and blinking of his eyes. He began to struggle with his reading; it was as if he could not see the words on the page, and he would squint and blink even more.   Reading had been a strength of his; now he was getting weaker by the day. Asa was continuing to thrive and get stronger in reading. He was passing Aiden up even though they had always been on a similar reading level.

Everyone at home would say, "Aiden, WHAT are you doing with your eyes?" I emailed his teacher and asked if he was having trouble seeing in class. Negative. I called the school nurse and asked if she would check his vision. She had just screened him a month or two prior. 20/20. It made no sense to me that he would have vision problems as my husband and I both had 20/20 vision. I was puzzled, and I made a note to myself to schedule an Optometry appointment after the Christmas break.

In January, I began to notice that Aiden was wetting the bed from time to time. We would sometimes hear Aiden get up to use the restroom within an hour of bedtime despite going potty just before being put in bed. He would still wet the bed despite this extra potty break. It was hard to detect as he would often just get up, use the restroom, and change his own clothes. I would catch it weekly maybe. It was easy to overlook and miss since he did change himself, and I worked nights two to four nights per week.

At the same time, he began to complain of stomach aches. He would come home from school and tell me how hungry he was. He was incredibly dramatic and over-reacted when I would tell him I was cooking or he had to wait. He would scream and stomp up the stairs if I told him dinner would be 10 minutes more. Or, he would fall to his knees and cry if I told him he was going to have to wait. His responses to the smallest slights were over-the-top. He would get aggressive and overly angry with his brothers. This Mom-of-the-Year would fuss at him for his behavior. I gave him lots of Tums.

By February, the bed-wetting was almost nightly. The cogs in my brain were starting to churn as I wondered why Aiden was wetting so much. At work, I was overseeing a "Biggest Loser" weight loss competition, so I was preparing the scale to take to work for the competition. On a Wednesday evening, seeing the scale, the twins wanted to weigh themselves. Asa weighed 56.5 pounds, and Aiden weighed 54 pounds. I was starting to think more about Aiden's symptoms, especially the bedwetting. I was adding it up in my mind, but once he got on the scale, THAT is when the red flag went up for me. Asa and Aiden only weighed an ounce apart at birth, and their growth and weight gain has always been pretty concordant. Never had they weighed more than a half-pound difference.

I must have made the strangest face when Aiden weighed because my husband immediately asked me what was wrong. I was putting two and two together. Bad behavior, bed-wetting, weight loss. When the twins left the room, I told him I was suspicious of Aiden and I would be calling the doctor in the morning. My heart was thumping hard inside my chest. I outlined the symptoms I noticed to him. "Uh oh" was all he said. In the meantime, I looked at Aiden's school memory book. On the first day of school (six months earlier) in August, he weighed 54 pounds. So, he had NO net weight gain in six months. It did not make sense. This guy is a BIG eater and had gained NO weight? It was impossible. My baby was starving to death despite being provided adequate nutrition.

I phoned the pediatrician on that Thursday morning and Aiden was worked into the schedule before lunch. By the time we saw the doctor, Aiden had not eaten in five to six hours. He was dumping glucose in his urine and his blood sugar was 140. Even though a blood sugar of 140 did not sound too alarming, I knew it should be much less after so long without food. A normal person would have a glucose almost half of that. I pointed out to his primary physician, Dr. H, that Aiden's weight was off and decreasing. The doctor was puzzled why Aiden had glucose in his urine but no ketones.

He scheduled Aiden for a 4-hour glucose tolerance test the next morning. I knew it was important, but it still was scary. I did not make it out of the office before I started crying because I did not want my baby to have to suffer through four separate venipunctures. As I mentioned, I had performed thousands of venipunctures in my life, and I have received my fair share. It is difficult to make it painless. I did not want him to suffer at all.

Aiden is super smart and understanding. I explained to him he was showing signs of Diabetes, and we needed to do some blood tests the next day. Because one of his grandfathers has Type Two Diabetes, he was familiar with the basics of the disease. Aiden had to fast, and I fasted with him. When we arrived at the laboratory the next morning, a 13-year-old was having his blood drawn and throwing a terrible fit. That did not comfort me very much. I was nervous Aiden would act the same or the teen's behavior would frighten Aiden. However, Aiden showed them how "big boys" act. He was nervous, but he sat still and tolerated every single blood draw. I was the only one who cried. I was so proud of him for being so brave!

To break our fast and celebrate his bravery, we had lunch at IHOP. Aiden ate his large pancake drenched in syrup and half of my food, too! He was starving!

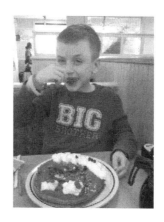

Aiden enjoying his IHOP lunch after fasting, Feb 17, 2012

At the time, I worked weekend nights. I went to work on Saturday and Sunday nights. I was pretty down and depressed. I barely spoke to my co-workers; I only told them something was going on and it had nothing to do with them. Fortunately, it was a slow weekend so I could just withdraw with my thoughts. I knew this was Diabetes, but I tried to find any other excuse for his symptoms. I came up empty. I did not sleep well at all the entire weekend. Sick. Sick with worry. I knew before I was told.

On February 20, 2012, a Monday morning, my co-workers and I stayed over at work for an IV pump class. About 10 minutes into the class, my cell phone rang. I recognized the pediatrician's office number. I grabbed my phone and stepped away to answer it. After I said, "Hello?" the nurse stated, "Mrs. Fuselier, Dr. H would like to speak to you." I knew. I knew then. The doctor RARELY wants to speak to someone over the phone! I went numb and tingly inside. I leaned against the wall so as not to fall. My world stopped turning in that moment. Time froze. Instantly, his life course was altered. Instantly, our lives were forever changed. And, instantly, I felt like my baby's life span had been shortened.

He told me Aiden's Glucose Tolerance Test (GTT) was abnormal. It was only 0815 and Dr. H had already consulted with Endocrinology. "It looks like you were right, Rhonda. He has Diabetes. He needs to go to the hospital right away. They are waiting for you. You did a good job, and you made a good catch. " That phone call was a defining moment in my life. My story forever changed. This was one of those rare occasions in my life when I did NOT want to be right! I asked what his GTT results were, and he said Aiden's glucose was over 400 the first two hours. God only knows how high his sugar was after our "celebratory" IHOP! I bet he was really dumping glucose and ketones in his urine after that meal! I am lucky I did not send him into a coma right then and there!

I grabbed my stuff and ran from the room. My fellow nurses looked at me like I was insane for my abrupt and tearful departure. I explained nothing, I just ran. I did not care about the class or the consequences for missing it. All I cared about was Aiden!

My husband had just reached the golf course with his friend. I called him, blubbering, and told him to meet me at home right away. The only description for what I did on the way home was blubber, bawl, and wail. I probably was not really fit to drive at that point. I could not think. I was jittery. I was scared to my core. He's my baby! I am the Mommy, dammit! It is my job to take care of him, keep him safe and fix things. I cannot fix this. ***Mommy can't fix it!***

Fortunately we only live five miles from my job. After arriving home, I packed a bag for each of us. I kept repeating to Jerry, "I am not leaving my baby! I am staying with him every minute!" I attempted to regain my composure. I could not lose it in front of Aiden.

I showered, washed my face, refreshed, and we got in the car to get Aiden out of school. He was surprised to see us. We had been keeping his teacher abreast of the situation, and we told her his diagnosis was confirmed and we had to take him to the hospital. The twins were in the same class that year. It was almost as hard to explain to his twin, Asa, that Aiden was sick and would be hospitalized while we left him alone without Aiden at school.

We explained to Aiden on the 20-minute drive to the hospital that his test results were bad and it confirmed Diabetes. He looked so scared and nervous, taxing the utmost limits of my now fragile composure. He was so tough. So brave. He never cried. The only thing he asked, which just twisted the knife that had just been jammed in my heart was, "Why me, Mommy?" I told him he was the one who was strong enough to deal with this. He was, but I was not sure if I was.

Cook Children's Medical Center was wonderful to Aiden. They were calm, and patient, and explained things to him on his level. He will still tell you today that they "treated me like a king". (Aiden got a Build-a-Bear, a Prayer Bear, a new pillow, a Mardi Gras parade with beads, and lots of treats and attention!) Remember, I had been up all night long at work the night before after sleeping poorly all weekend. Now, I was up all day, too! I think shock and adrenaline kept me awake. They deferred the primary Diabetes education until the next day so I could perhaps comprehend and retain what was being taught. The first day was spent with more testing, stabilizing Aiden metabolically, and initiating insulin therapy. Since the changes are gradual, I never realized how ill Aiden looked until he was restored to health.

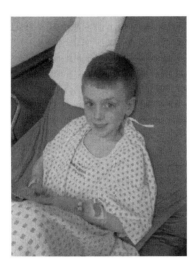

Aiden upon admission, Feb 20, 2012

My husband stayed with us until it was time to be home for the other boys getting out of school. He took care of the business at home and then brought Aiden's brothers to see him. Asa especially really needed to see Aiden. My son, Kyle, came into the room and abruptly stepped out for a few minutes. He later told me it broke his heart to see Aiden sick lying in a hospital bed. He regained his strength and then returned. Aiden was happy to see his brothers and show them the playroom. I was happy to just have my husband back, one more time, to hold me.

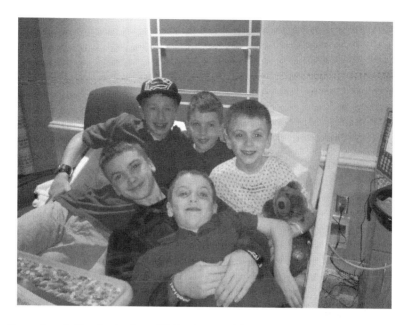

From top left, clockwise: (Kyle, Jace, Aiden, and Gage holding Asa)
visiting Aiden in the hospital.

After Jerry left for the afternoon, my friend stopped by the house to grab a small bag I wanted that Jerry had prepared for me. She brought it to me and visited with us. It had another shirt and my MP3 player. I needed my "dope", my Bon Jovi music. I did not check the bag for awhile. When I did, the tears started all over again. Jerry had slipped a note in the bag that said, "You're an amazing wife and an even better Mommy. I'm thankful for you every day. I love you".

We made a point to call close family members and our best friends before we posted anything on Facebook about Aiden. It was difficult to even say the words as saying it made it more real. If I did not have to say it, maybe I could wake up from this nightmare. My phone rang and the text messages flooded in. Our family and closest friends were worried about us and Aiden. My parents came to visit, too, to make sure their grandbaby (and daughter) was okay.

Around 9 pm, I had been awake at least 30 hours, and I finally got to sleep. After sleeping about one hour, I was awakened to the sound of the nurses trying to rouse Aiden. They were calling his name and he was unresponsive to them. Of course, I jumped up, and started calling Aiden's name to get him to drink juice. His sugar was low. 34. Too much insulin. He recognized my voice. He responded only to me, but the vacant look in his big blue eyes and the way they darted back and forth haphazardly only made me cry again. Needless to say, I only dozed during the night, frequently jumping up to check on him. It made for one of the longest nights of my life. It was a precursor to how many nights would be for the foreseeable future.

The next day was spent learning. We were visited by the Certified Diabetes Nurse Educator (CDE), the Social Worker, the Nutritionist and the Endocrinologist. I did not care much for the Social Worker visit as I feel she wanted me to discuss my very raw emotions and feelings in front of my innocent child. I had not fully processed them myself. I politely told her I was coping, but I would not be discussing adult emotions and issues in front of Aiden. The rest of the Diabetes team was great for us!

We spent so much time learning, not yet knowing it was only the tip of the iceberg. We were also trying to figure out the right amount of insulin for Aiden and helping him learn, too. It was sad to watch my non-medical, very technical husband have to learn to jab a needle into the arm of his son. Jerry had to learn how to prick Aiden's finger, and I had to demonstrate my proficiency at such tasks, despite my resume. We poked each other's fingers for practice. Jerry did not bleed easily with the lancet device on the lowest one or two setting, so I cranked it up to seven, the maximum setting. Um, needless to say, he bled...and felt it! He was not very impressed with me over that one, and he still reminds me about it! I later asked him if he was scared. "I don't like it, but if I don't do it, my kid dies. What choice do I have?" I am so fortunate to have an intelligent, willing and able partner who is right there beside me in managing Diabetes care.

Aiden's second night in the hospital was much smoother. As I put him to bed, he hugged me. Long, firm, wouldn't let go. Then, he kissed me multiple times and said, "I love you, Mommy!" I just held my baby, thankful he was alive. Although this diagnosis sucked, I was so grateful it was not a terminal diagnosis. I fought back tears as I continued to try hard not to cry in front of Aiden. I did not want him to be frightened by my tears or feel responsible for making me sad. In another day or time, I would have lost him. 100 years ago, this would have been a death sentence!

We worked on insulin, counting carbs, and calculating doses. It was lots of work. Even for an educated professional in the medical field, there was tons of learning. With every meal, we had to count what he had eaten and approximate what percentage he had eaten, and then add it all up. Figuring the right amount of insulin was a quick test of our math skills! Nursing school did not prepare me for the ins and outs of day-to-day diabetes management!

We spent three days and two nights in the hospital. Two-and-a-half days learning how to keep him alive; it hardly seemed long enough. Prior to our discharge, I sent Jerry to the store to load the house up with free snacks and other supplies. We came home on Wednesday evening. Home to a new life, adjusting to a new normal. Blood sugars, meters, strips, syringes, alcohol, Lantus and Humalog. We had our Pink Panther Book to guide us, and Aiden had his JDRF Hope Backpack with Rufus the Diabetes Bear.

The following day, Aiden went back to school. I met with the school nurse briefly and gave her basic supplies, our care plan, and insulin. I spent the entire day filling prescriptions, making emergency kits and supply kits for each grandmother and the school nurse. I returned later to meet again with the nurse and give her more supplies. I was greeted by the school counselor who asked me about scheduling a meeting for a "504 Plan". It was overwhelming, a foreign language. I could only deal with one thing at a time! Getting organized was Step One and critical. That is just how my brain works. The day was quite overwhelming, especially the $600 bill just to leave the pharmacy. Six Hundred Dollars. But, how do you put a price on your baby's life?

I felt like I had lost control and security because I could not fix this. I was not born to be a pancreas, but suddenly I was catapulted into that role…just to keep my baby alive. I did not ask for the job. I did not apply for the job. And, I cannot quit the job.

Chapter Two: Type One Vs. Type Two Diabetes

Just a little background information.

Type One Diabetes

An autoimmune disease is: An illness that occurs when the body tissues are attacked by its own immune system. The immune system is a complex organization within the body that is designed normally to "seek and destroy" invaders of the body, including infectious agents. Patients with autoimmune diseases frequently have unusual antibodies circulating in their blood that target their own body tissues. *(medterms.com)* Autoimmune Diseases include such things as Multiple Sclerosis, Lupus, Celiac Disease, Psoriasis, and Rheumatoid Arthritis.

Type One Diabetes is an autoimmune disease.

Type 1 Diabetes (T1D) is an autoimmune disease in which a person's pancreas stops producing insulin, a hormone that enables people to get energy from food. It occurs when the body's immune system attacks and destroys the insulin-producing cells in the pancreas, called beta cells. While its causes are not yet entirely understood, scientists believe that both genetic factors and environmental triggers are involved. **Its onset has nothing to do with diet or lifestyle.** There is nothing you can do to prevent T1D, and at present, nothing you can do to get rid of it. *(JDRF.org)* Most people who develop Type 1 are otherwise healthy.

Type One Diabetes plays no favorites. It does not discriminate on the basis of age, color, creed, religion or economic status. I have heard of people being diagnosed as young as 6 months old and as old as age 33. Most T1D patients are diagnosed before their early 20's.

Type Two Diabetes

Type 2 Diabetes is one of the two major types of diabetes and is more common in the general public. It is a metabolic (not autoimmune) disorder. It is the type in which the beta cells of the pancreas produce insulin, but the body is unable to use it effectively because the cells of the body are resistant to the action of insulin and/or they don't produce enough insulin. Although this type of diabetes may not carry the same risk of death from ketoacidosis, it otherwise involves many of the same risks of complications as does Type One Diabetes (in which there is a lack of insulin entirely). The aim of treatment is to normalize the blood glucose in an attempt to prevent or minimize complications. People with T2D may experience marked hyperglycemia, but most do not require insulin injections. In fact, 80% of all people with T2D can be treated with diet, exercise, and, if need be, oral hypoglycemia agents (drugs taken by mouth to lower the blood sugar). Over time with progression of the disease, insulin use may become necessary.

Type 2 Diabetes requires good dietary control including the restriction of calories, lowered consumption of simple carbohydrates and fat with increased consumption of complex carbohydrates and fiber. Regular aerobic exercise is also an important method for treating both types of diabetes since it decreases insulin resistance and helps burn excessive glucose. Regular exercise also may help lower blood lipids and reduce some effects of stress, both of which are important in treating diabetes and preventing complications (*medterms.com)*

Type 2 Diabetes can have a hereditary link, and it can also be closely linked to lifestyle. A pancreas is only designed to care for a certain sized body, and when you tax its limits, it cannot keep up. Here is my little analogy: Your pancreas is the car's engine; gasoline is the carb (fuel). I equate this to overloading a trailer and trying to drag it behind your car. Your car CAN go, but very inefficiently. It does not process the fuel correctly. If you remove the load, then the car can again function normally. If you drag that load too long and do not maintain the car, it can and will be permanently damaged. My boys' engine died, so it does not matter what we do, it will not start again. It cannot use its fuel without help.

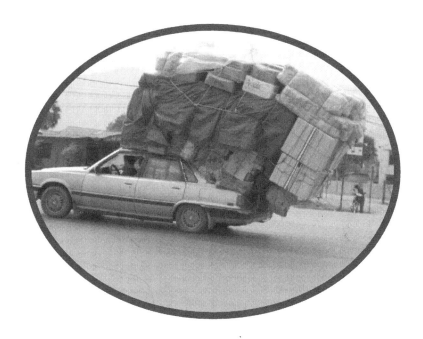

Treatments and alleged cures

There are a lot of books out there about Diabetes miracle cures and treatments. Most of these refer to Type 2 Diabetes and will NOT help with T1D. Trust me, if it would, I would have tried it already....multiple times. If cinnamon would help, I would have already made them eat spoonfuls of it. If honey would help, I would have injected it into their veins already. (Instead, they need lots of insulin to cover the carbs in honey!) If an alkaline diet would help, I would have already given them an Alka-Seltzer enema. (Not sure that would cover it, but it sounds good!) And, if the leaves of some exotic plant would cure them, I would travel barefoot to the distant land, sing and dance naked while I picked the leaves, then they would drink the tea daily. Unfortunately for them, none of that will take away the attack on their tiny pancreases. I wish it would. Mommy would do anything to take it away and fix it. Currently, the only treatment for Type One Diabetes is insulin injections.

Signs of Hypoglycemia (Low Blood Sugar)

Low blood sugar is a glucose level that is below the normal range, usually 70 mg/dl. Hypoglycemia can be caused by too much or too rapid of an absorption of insulin, heavy exercise, not eating enough or illness. Signs of low blood sugar include dizziness, confusion, behavior changes, nausea, extreme hunger, irritability, inability to concentrate. The only way to remedy this is to provide carbohydrates. We commonly offer carbs in the form of glucose tablets, juice, candy, and/or chocolate milk.

Hypoglycemia can be severe and lead to shock, convulsion, loss of consciousness and/or death. If it becomes this severe, Glucagon has to be administered and 911 called. Fortunately (knock on wood), we have not seen a severe low thus far. We have seen some pretty impressive low blood sugars that warrant immediate treatment (in the 30s and 40s), but none so far have made him lose consciousness (besides the one almost in the hospital). We have been very fortunate. A T1D parent has to know what signs their child shows and recognize them. Aiden will often say he feels hungry, confused or he has "shaky legs". There is not one number that will send a person into severe hypoglycemia. Every person is different, and every day is different.

Signs of Hyperglycemia (High Blood Sugar)

Hyperglycemia occurs when a person has too much glucose in the blood that is not able to be used by the cells due to inadequate insulin. It can be caused by stress, illness, insufficient amount of or poorly absorbed insulin, eating more than usual or not enough exercise. The way to remedy hyperglycemia is with exercise, hydration and more insulin. Unlike hypoglycemia, high blood sugar does not put the T1D patient in immediate danger; however, hyperglycemia is what causes bodily damage and organ dysfunction over time.

Complications resulting from hyperglycemia include diabetic ketoacidosis (DKA), amputations, blindness, nerve damage, heart disease, kidney failure, and death. Diabetic ketoacidosis occurs when the body burns fat and muscle for energy because it cannot access the glucose in the blood. The breakdown of fats leads to ketones in the blood which causes an acidotic state in the body; too many ketones are basically poisonous. This will cause the person to go into a coma. Unfortunately, this is how many people discover they are diabetic. And, poor management will lead to rehospitalizations due to DKA.

When a diabetic is hyperglycemic, he has frequent urination (because sugar in the blood is a diuretic); extreme thirst (because he/she is dehydrated from the frequent urination); blurry vision; stomach pain; hunger (because the body thinks it's starving since it can't access the glucose); nausea and vomiting; weight loss (because the body is burning fat for energy and dehydrated); inability to concentrate; fruity smelling breath; and, behavior changes including irritability and aggressiveness.

Hindsight is 20/20. When Aiden got on the scale, it all started adding up. His bad behavior, his bed-wetting, his weight, his frequent stomach aches. Later I figured out his squinting was also from the T1D. His vision was blurry, but he did not know how to articulate that. Once on insulin, problem solved. Today, when his sugar is too high or he has a particularly heavy meal, he'll complain of stomach pains and his attitude stinks! At "Memaw's" house recently, he had an outburst with his brother. She said, "Well, his sugar must be high!" And, it was!

The doctor assured us that Aiden was young enough that his state upon admission did not cause permanent damage. But, that little Mommy-guilt piece of me wonders. I wonder every time he is too high if my failures in managing his blood sugar are causing permanent harm or damage to him. Parents, children, and Diabetes alike have good days and bad days, but with good control, complications can be avoided, delayed or minimized.

Chapter Three: A Family Affair

As I mentioned, as a blended family, Jerry and I have seven children total. At the time of Aiden's diagnosis, Jerry's daughter Maegen was 22 and living on her own. Maegen is the only child who never lived with us full-time. She was nine when we met. My daughter, Courtney, was 20 and engaged to be married. She lived on-campus in college about an hour away from home. Jerry's son, Gage, was 14 and we have had custody of him for over six years. My son, Kyle, was a month shy of 14. Our first son, Jace, was eight, and our twins were seven. With our girls gone, there is a lot of testosterone in my home.

We had been talking to our boys about Aiden's care, and like I mentioned, they came to see him in the hospital and to bring us home from the hospital. In addition, my daughter was away in college and home on the breaks and weekends. We kept her abreast of the situation via phone and text. I tried not to worry her too much so she could focus on her studies. She was eager to get home on the weekend after diagnosis to see Aiden and bring him a special prize to make him feel better. This disease instantly became not just Aiden's disease, but everyone's disease.

We immediately made the rule that if Aiden could not have it, nobody could. This rule, we felt, showed solidarity and fairness and would help Aiden adjust any limitations of his disease. Fortunately for us, we already maintained a relatively healthy diet. Whole grains, fruits, vegetables, lean meats and skim milk. We limited junk, excess sugar, and processed foods. Fast food was the exception, not the rule, and restaurant dining was infrequent due to the extreme cost of feeding that many people outside the home. I already bought the children diet non-caffeinated flavored sodas (and limited them to one per day) because they were too rowdy with too much sugar or caffeine on board! Water was the encouraged drink of choice. Not too many adjustments had to be made.

ALL boys got to have their fingers poked so they would know what Aiden felt. ALL boys were taught the signs of hypoglycemia including confusion, irritability, shakiness, and extreme hunger. It was made abundantly clear that nobody at any point in time would ignore these signs in Aiden. It became comical because when they would fight, like brothers do, and Aiden would get upset, we heard someone yell, "Mommy! You need to check Aiden's sugar! He's being a jerk!"

The teenage boys and our daughter were taught how to check Aiden's blood sugar and read the first few chapters of the Pink Panther book so that they could understand the disease and help respond in an emergency. They were taught the "Rule of 15s" (Treat a low with 15 g of carbohydrates and repeat the test in 15 minutes) and how to treat and recheck if Aiden was low. It seems a big burden to place on another child, but anyone who has or cares for a diabetic knows that you need all eyes open all the time. Mommy has to shower, use the restroom and sleep occasionally! Whenever needed, tender-hearted Kyle is usually the one who takes the reins on this. Everyone knows how to count carbs, read labels, and they remind Aiden to take his insulin or check his sugar. Besides providing for his safety, involving all siblings made them feel involved and fostered a supportive atmosphere.

Paying for and managing Aiden's disease took a toll on my abilities to participate in planning and funding my daughter's wedding. We had already helped pay for quite a few things, and she was relying on her father and her grandparents to help, too. I had intended to help pay for a few more things, but I was unable. I explained to her, "I can use this money to keep your brother alive, or I can pay for extra wedding stuff." The choice was obvious to both of us. She found frugal ways to get what she wanted and saved and used every dime she and her fiancé made in order to have a lovely ceremony.

My time to help her was also limited. We were on a high deductible health plan because we really only used our insurance coverage for monthly medications and wellness examinations. We never dreamed this would happen. So, we were left paying a tremendous amount of money out of pocket. We had to pay for prescriptions, supplies, hospitalizations, and physician bills. In addition to those funds going to medical care, my time to help my daughter was also diminished as I had to work plenty of extra shifts to earn the money to cover the bills.

Aiden and Asa were ring bearers in the wedding. They were so cute and handsome. At rehearsal and prior to the wedding, we had to stop and check a blood sugar. We had to carb up if needed. I was so worried he would feel low (or go hypoglycemic) during the wedding and detract from the ceremony. Fortunately, everything went off without a hitch as far as Diabetes is concerned.

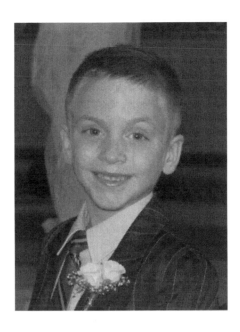

Ring Bearer Aiden, June 2012

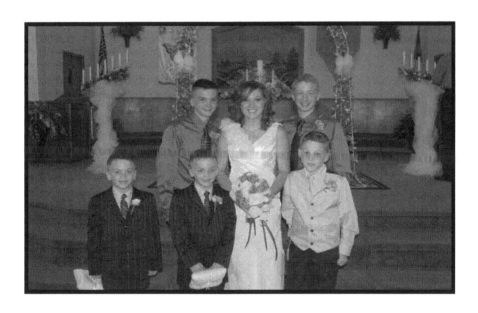

Courtney and her brothers at her wedding, June 2012

After my daughter was married in June, she wanted her brothers to spend the night at her apartment. She made a point to then learn insulin injections, insulin-to-carb ratios (I:C), etc. It pained her to stab her baby brother, but she wanted to spend that time with him. We were only a phone call away. I could not deny Aiden this precious time with his sister. If everyone else got to do it, so should he. She did a great job each visit, but right on cue, he would go low and/or spike high each time just to make her nervous. More than one night we were on the phone with her guiding her how to handle a high or low sugar. She experienced Diabetes sleep deprivation early on!

I made a box for each grandmother that included some basic supplies (syringes, strips, alcohol) and emergency hypoglycemia provisions. I gave each grandmother the Pink Panther book to read in addition to copies of handouts listing signs of hypoglycemia and hyperglycemia. I made a file on my computer that outlined most aspects of Aiden's care including emergency phone numbers, how to respond to hypoglycemia, and which insulin to give when and why. Furthermore, we bought Aiden a cool Transformers lunchbox and made his "Diabetes kit". Inside are Glucagon, low blood sugar remedies, and other basic supplies to go anywhere we go with him.

When we decided to begin insulin pump therapy, both grandmothers attended class with us so they could fully understand the ins and outs of pumping. Without a doubt, we had great family support brimming with love and concern for Aiden. Jerry's mother and step-father typically take the kids for an overnight visit every other weekend. Connie ("Memaw") wasn't scared and refused to let that change due to Diabetes. She defers to our decisions and judgments; she documents carbs, blood sugars and insulin; she has been wonderful to make sure Aiden feels no different due to his disease. I work nights, so I am always a phone call or text away if she has any questions any time of day or night. My mother babysits when we have dates and comes and spends time at our home when we take vacations. She is a nurse, too, and she never blinked about taking care of Aiden. I do not know what we would do without this respite.

Since Aiden's diagnosis, we made sure each boy checked their blood sugars periodically. We especially monitored twin Asa and full-brother Jace. They always looked good. Until one day in August....

Family Affair

It was 1963. I remember it well. We lived in San Diego, CA. It was the year The Beatles came to America. My family moved that summer to Van Nuys, CA into a two bedroom apartment. There was my dad, mom, little sister and two older brothers. Within the first two weeks of the school year, I started getting sick. My mother thought it was the flu. It was so bad so quick I left school (the 5th Grade). I missed almost that whole year as it turned out, but I'll get to that a little later.

Sometimes I would sit in the bathtub for hours, not because I was a clean kid. OH No! I would stay in there so I could drink the water because I was so thirsty. Then I would throw up in the toilet and start over again. Some nights I would wake up and be so hungry I would eat anything I could get my hands on. As it turned out my drinking the water was from high sugars and the eating was from low sugars. Over one night I ate a complete devils food cake by myself. I suffered a lot the next day.

Finally it all came to this: My Dad, mom, older brother, little sister and I went out to eat dinner. I even remember the name of the restaurant, Van De Kamps. This has meaning later on in this statement. I was not feeling very well, as you could imagine. I decided to get up go to the restroom and drink from the sink (again, high sugar level). When I excused myself and stood up, I fainted.

I was rushed to Northridge Hospital that was in the same parking lot as the restaurant. I lay in the hallway for hours until a doctor came in and saw me there. She asked my mother why I was there. Of course, my mother had no idea and could not articulate what was wrong; this had been going on for so long.

The doctors name was Rothchild. She ordered me into the Emergency Room for evaluation. This is where it gets a little strange for me. Some people believe me and some do not, but here it is. I went into a deep sleep. My sugar was so high it did not register on the equipment that was available at the time. I *actually watched from above as several doctors tried to revive me. It seemed like a long time but I found out later it was only a few minutes. Anyways, I was stabilized and came back from wherever that place was.*

I woke to hear Dr. Rothchild fill my mother and brother in on my situation. I heard Dr. Rothchild say, "Your child has Diabetes. He was so bad we almost lost him! We are trying to stabilize him, but I cannot say at this time what the outcome will be."

I wondered how my mother was accepting that her ten-year-old may not survive. She lost a son early in her marriage and now possibly another. To what? What was this Diabetes sickness? Two days later I regained consciousness. I was lying in the hospital trying to figure out why I was there and who all these people were. Why do I have tubes in my arm? Why aren't they feeding me real food? Questions and more questions.

Finally my doctor appeared. She told me what I had, but I did not understand. This was almost fifty years ago and the medical world knew nowhere near as much as now. I was hospitalized for two weeks. It was scary the first week, but then I became the nurses' favorite. They brought me toys (it was my birthday) and spoiled me rotten, but then put me to work folding towels and delivering food to other rooms. I found out later they were testing me to see how I would react to the medications.

I finally went home after two weeks. It was tough for a long time. I was taken to the hospital numerous times for high and low sugars. Somewhere along the line, with the love and twenty-four-hour coverage and care by my mother, I made my way. There is no doubt that Type One Diabetes is a family affair!

Fifty years ago, when I went to the doctor for anything they would take a blood sample and send it to the lab. I would find out a week later what my level was. Well, as we know now your level can change in minutes...Now we know in seconds! Look how far we've come in fifty years. It's amazing.

Remember that statement about the restaurant in the same parking lot as the hospital? The medical building where I currently visit my endocrinologist is on the same corner that restaurant once was. Weird. Also Dr. Rothchild told my mother and brother that there was little chance that I would survive to be thirteen. I have lived with that statement on my mind for the last forty-nine years.

Family really matters in managing this disease! It was the love and courage of my mother, my first wife, Jaci, and my wife of 30 years and soul-mate, Debra that pulled me through all those hard and scary times. Now here I am, retired, living my life as well as I can, and trying to do the right thing for my health.

Although I am the only sibling with Type One Diabetes, three of my older brothers have since been diagnosed with Type Two Diabetes. I hoped that neither of my sons would develop this disease like me, and they have not. However, not too long ago my oldest son called to tell me my grandson was diagnosed with Type One Diabetes. I was devastated and somehow felt responsible. I cried. A few months later, his twin was diagnosed with Type One Diabetes. I was devastated again. Somehow I never really thought that would happen. I was wrong. I guess I just thought all would be OK. I would give anything for that to not have happened, however if we look back at how it was when I went through it all, maybe we can be glad that so much has been learned since then. Most importantly, how can we find a cure so no more children have to experience what we did?

By the way, Dr Rothchild, "I'll be sixty years old soon. I'm glad to say 'you were wrong'!"

John Johnson, Sr.

Type One Diabetic since age 10

Biological Grandfather of Asa & Aiden Fuselier

Chapter Four: Double Whammy

When Aiden was diagnosed, one of the first questions we asked the Endocrinologist was about Asa.   What was his risk of also developing T1D since he is genetically the same person as Aiden? Can we use cells from Asa to help Aiden? (By the way, only cadaver transplants are conducted, so we decided we would not kill Asa to cure Aiden). We were told there was about a 10% chance of Asa also developing Diabetes. We were falsely reassured by that number. We crossed our fingers. We hoped Asa would dodge that bullet.

Once home, I did more research, and I was in discussion with TrialNet about having all of Jerry's biological sons tested for T1D antibodies. I learned that Asa had a 10% chance of developing Diabetes in the first year of his twin's diagnosis, and a 50% chance over the course of his lifetime. The odds were lower than that for non-twin siblings, which in our family would be Gage and Jace.

Asa is definitely the more sensitive, fearful and tender twin. We used to tease him, pretending we thought he was Aiden and act like we were going to give him a shot or check his sugar. He would resist, flinch, and scream, "I'M NOT AIDEN! I DON'T HAVE DIABETES!" Someone asked me once if we had ever mixed them up like that. I responded there was no way in Hell Asa would let that happen! ☺ We checked Asa's sugar periodically, and he was always very reluctant and whiny when we wanted to check. His numbers looked consistently normal. At his routine check-up appointment with Dr. Halpenny in June or July of 2012, we discussed Asa's risk, how we checked him occasionally, and how we would consult with the Endocrinologist in August about having Asa tested. Aiden's next appointment was in late August.

On August 3, 2012, Aiden came downstairs two hours after lunch claiming he "felt low". Oddly, Asa said, "Check my sugar, too!" Remember, this is the same kid who resisted, fought and whined every time we suggested he check his blood glucose. I checked Aiden and corrected his low. Seizing the chance to check on Asa without a fight, I tested his blood sugar. He was over 200....two hours *after* lunch. Crap. My heart sank. I looked at him, back and the meter and back at him again. I could not believe my eyes. A repeat test revealed the same result. My world stopped turning again. Time froze. All the not-so-old emotions surrounding Aiden's diagnosis flooded over me. A new set of emotions consumed me. And, so it began.

Trying to add it all up, I put Asa on the scale, and he was down to 55 pounds (remember, he was 56.5 in February). I had to work Friday, Saturday, and Sunday nights. My husband and I checked Asa in the morning and before every meal throughout the weekend. His morning fasting glucose was normal each morning, but his level would not venture below 200 all day before or after meals. Every time I saw a high number the entire weekend, I felt like the knife was being stabbed into my heart a little deeper. I felt like I was spiraling down a drain emotionally.

I retreated again at work. Depressed. Crying. Sad. Now two babies? Really? How is this fair? Again, I tried to find an excuse for the hyperglycemia, and I came up empty. He was not ill. He was not on any medications. His diet was unchanged. It is theorized that the T1D autoimmune response is triggered by a virus. With Aiden, I blamed that flu vaccine. I was convinced. Now, my beautiful, perfect, healthy baby Asa was sick. I had nothing or nobody to blame.

After working all night the night before, on August 6, 2012, a Monday morning, I called the pediatrician's office. I told the nurse my suspicions and requested an appointment. They were crazy busy because people were doing last minute pre-school physicals. She wanted to see him the next day. I begged her to work us in in the afternoon, and I promised I would not complain about the wait. We got an appointment for 4 pm. I got some sleep, and I waited for the time for the appointment, continuing to check his blood glucose. Jerry came home early to care for the other boys while I was gone. I brought Asa and our sheet of blood sugars to the pediatrician's office. They obtained a urine specimen from Asa. Again, I knew before I was told.

Dr. H came in and just gave me a look. His face said it all. "I am sorry, Rhonda. It looks like you have another one". Damn it, I was right again. I caught it early. Yippee. I held it together this time, barely. I spent the whole weekend crying already. Asa was spilling glucose and ketones into his urine. He called Aiden's endocrinologist, they consulted, and I had to take Asa to the hospital, too. We went home, packed bags, and told the other boys.

Aiden was scared for Asa, but sort of happy, too. Now, somebody was like him. Now, he was not alone. I thank my lucky stars every day that if this was our destiny, I am glad Aiden went first. He is the tougher and braver twin. I think Asa handled his diagnosis so well because he had watched Aiden for the last five months. He was somewhat excited to go to the hospital and get the same goodies that Aiden received, and it was not so scary and foreign to him. So much for our 10% odds.

Asa was much less ill upon diagnosis, so we only spent 24 hours in the hospital. The same trail of people came into the room. Diabetes Nurse, Social Worker, Nutritionist. This visit was not so much about us being educated as it was about getting Asa metabolically stable and allowing him the education he needed and the transition from wellness to lifelong disease. He got his Prayer Bear, his JDRF Rufus backpack, and his Build-a-Bear. Jerry brought the other boys to see Asa in the hospital, too.

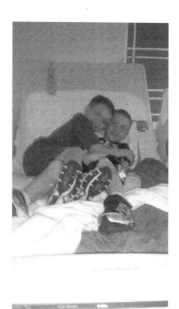

Aiden hugging Asa in the hospital, August 7, 2012

On Tuesday night, we went home to another more complicated, more intense, new normal. Two meters, two doses of insulin, two blood sugar checks, and two times the amount of supplies with the added complexity of trying not to mix up which boy was being tested or treated. Yet again, something Mommy can't fix.

I insisted upon Asa's diagnosis that each boy have the exact same insulin, exact same supplies and prescriptions, and the same endocrinology appointments. With five boys in the house, I already chase my tail enough trying to keep up. I did not need to chase my tail trying to keep up with separate Diabetes plans and supplies, too! A dog can only chase its tail so long before it just collapses.

So, here we are. Two boys. Our babies, our twins. Two Type One Diabetes Diagnoses. We had statistically low odds to have identical twins, and we got twins. They were the statistical outliers as identical twins in that they did not share or have bordering placentas. We were given statistically low odds for both boys to have this disease. They broke the rules at every turn.

At our first Endocrinology appointment for Asa (which was the same as Aiden's second visit….all visits the same), our Endocrinologist told us that the boys tested positive for all three T1D antibodies. Most kids have one or two. My little "Rule Breakers" have all three. Triple attack and assault on those little pancreases. Life is fair, right?

The boys are funny now. They compare blood sugars at testing time. They walk to the school nurse together. They worry about each other if something is off. Twin bonds are incredible to watch, unique and special, but I think theirs is deeper and more intense. They are in this together. And, being identical (quite identical) twins has led to some mishaps and blunders on our parts.

Chapter Five: Emotional Roller-Coaster

"I lost all faith in my God, and His religion, too.
I told the angels they could sing their song to someone new.
I lost all trust in my friends; I watched my heart turn to stone.
I thought that I was left to walk this wicked world alone..."

It is as much a loss for a parent to have a child diagnosed with Type One Diabetes as it is for the child. I had my babies at age 30, and my full intention is to live to be 100. I have no intention of burying my babies, but realistically, I know my babies' life spans could be shortened dramatically if their disease is not managed well. As I have grown and learned and researched, I know that they may have just as long and good a life as any non-diabetic child, especially since such a focus is put on healthy living as a mainstay for diabetic control. Better treatments are coming and a cure is on the horizon. Despite all that, I cannot just take it and run. On a day to day basis I cope, but sometimes, it just gets to me. I get angry. I get depressed. Frustrated. Disgusted. We have good days and bad days. As I am sure any D-mom does, I have run the gamut of emotions. I think (and hope) these are all normal.

Anger and Resentment

First and foremost, it is not fair. I had a healthy pregnancy. I stayed on bedrest, per doctor's orders, in order to carry my babies as long as possible. I almost exclusively breastfed my twins for 8 months. I exercise, and I make sure my children are physically active. I preach and practice healthy eating. Perfect? No, but overall, pretty healthy. I take my kids to the doctor routinely. They get regular check-ups at the dentist. They've received all their immunizations on schedule. I've done everything known to man that is supposed to statistically lower their risk of developing T1D, yet they still got it. It makes me angry. Actually, it pisses me off!

I see people who do everything wrong in their pregnancies. (Drugs, smoking, poor eating habits, never drinking water, alcohol use). I see ignorant or desperate people put substances in their babies' bottles like soda and Kool-aid. I see children whose medical care and immunization schedule is neglected. And, I see parents who abuse their own bodies and the bodies of their children on a regular basis. Poor eating. Junk food. Fast food. Inactivity. Obesity. But, MY children have Diabetes?! Granted, I do not wish it on anyone, but it does make a Mommy who has done it all right pretty resentful. While sitting in the pediatrician's waiting room after my boys were diagnosed, I saw a large rotund man walk his equally rotund 200+ pound 12-yr-old into the examination room. Logically, I know my children are ultimately healthier than that unfortunate child, but it still fertilizes the seeds of anger and resentment. Trust me, I KNOW this is not a disease of lifestyle. I am not saying my feelings are perfectly rational. They are what they are. But, if someone has to have the disease, should it not be the one who is messing everything up?

In my job, we get the occasional T1D patient, and sometimes I just want to scream at them. Do they not understand or care? My name is not Jesus and I am not here to judge; I have to remember that. However, I become so frustrated knowing I try so hard to manage my boys' blood sugars and these ladies are lackadaisical about their care. Chips, fast food, missed insulin, and completely unfazed by glucose levels over 200. Now, as a pregnant woman, they are impacting the health of their fetuses to boot. Fetuses subjected to uncontrolled blood glucoses are prone to heart defects, large size which can lead to birth injuries and unstable blood sugars of their own after their birth. I am left wondering if their parents did not try hard in managing their care or if the patient got lazy and complacent when it was their time to take the reins.

Mommy Guilt

You never feel as if you are doing the right thing as a parent, and you wonder if the care and guidance you are providing is hitting or missing the mark with your children. I have read that a good mother is certain she is screwing up! With T1D, this guilt and these fears are compounded. Now, I have to wonder not only about parenting in general, but also managing this disease in two little guys. I was not born a pancreas, but now I have to act as two. It is a full-time job, and I am working overtime. And, when things do not go according to plan, the feeling of failure and disappointment is overwhelming.

Mommy guilt plagues me because I feel the sheer amount of time, worry, and attention I spend managing two diabetics is taking time away from the other non-diabetic children. Unintentionally, the twins and Diabetes commandeer a large chunk of my time. I have to be very conscientious to carve out a piece of time for each of them, but there are days I am left with very little to offer.

Across Aiden's care, his Hemoglobin A1C was steadily declining to a near-normal level. We check it every 3 months. As time progressed, we learned Aiden's habits, tweaked his dosages, and researched Diabetes care ad nauseum. In November, two months after we started pump therapy, I thought things were going very well. I was feeling pretty confident that I had the upper hand and things were well under control. I keep diligent records, average blood sugars daily and weekly, and constantly analyze numbers, rates, and dosages.

Three months after diagnosis, Asa was down 1.2 points. Great! Aiden's HgbA1C had declined the last two visits, so I waited eagerly to hear Aiden's number. It was 0.6 points **higher** than the last quarter's A1C. I was shocked. That was not the result I expected! Instantly I felt like a failure. My eyes welled up with tears. I tried to hold back, but I just could not. Against my wishes and much to my chagrin, I cried right there in the CDE's office. That number just told me that my hard work, getting up in the night (sometimes multiple times), adjusting, testing, and trying my hardest....it was not good enough. Diabetes and perfectionism do not mix. In that moment, Diabetes kicked me in the face and showed me who was boss. Apparently, it is not me!

I cried again when the Endocrinologist came into the room to talk about my boys and their care. All I could say was, "It's not supposed to go UP! The same or lower, NOT higher! That's it!" She reassured me that I was doing well. Aiden's growing. He is quickly exiting the "honeymoon phase" of this disease. The A1C is used as a gauge to guide care and is not a report card. We adjusted some numbers for Aiden. My boys looked so worried about why I was crying which was precisely why I try so hard not to cry in front of them. When the physician left the room, the questions came.

Aiden: Mommy, why are you crying?

Me: Because, baby, that number was not what I wanted it to be. (How can I phrase this in a way he understands without unloading too much on him?)

Aiden: Is it bad?

Me: No, it is not bad; I just thought it would be better. Mommy wants everything just right for you, and I try hard.

Aiden: It's ok, Mommy. It's not like I'm dying or anything. (Ever the pragmatist)

Obviously, kids live day-to-day and move on. As long as he was not dying, Aiden was alright. But as a Mommy, I internalize it and I look around corners. Right now, he just does not understand how much stock I put into this serious job of being his pancreas. He cannot fathom or understand how I felt like I failed him. He does not understand how much I love him. The A1C tells everyone how well Diabetes is being managed this quarter. Unless being a pancreas is your job, you cannot understand how even though it is "not a report card", I feel like it is. This straight-A student does not like to get failing grades.

I am a sap when it comes to being upset. I can hold it together unless I talk to my mom or my husband. I knew I would break down crying in front of my boys again, so I planned to delay my call to Jerry until I got the boys back to school and calmed down. But, he beat me to the punch. He called while we were still in the exam room waiting for the nurse to bring in the flu vaccines. I just busted out crying. He thought something was *terribly* wrong. Once my speech was perceptible and he understood why I was upset, he was relieved and reassuring. Still. I only want what is good for them. Now, I have made a deal with myself to be happy with a range instead of expecting a particular number (or less). With my continual analysis of numbers, I can semi-predict what the A1C will look like.

To add insult to injury, Aiden's Hemoglobin A1C rose **again** the next quarter. I shook my head in disgust because I knew I had worked very hard to bring it down or keep it steady, but it did not work. I did stave off tears this time. To remedy the situation, I focused on a couple of areas to try to adjust to bring the A1C back down. We changed our meter and conducted multiple bolus and basal tests. We also began pre-dosing. But, before we could see if our efforts were successful, the boys had to see the Ophthalmologist. While doing their exam, the Optical Tech asked questions about the boys' Diabetes. When I told him what Aiden's latest A1C was, he made a humph sound and left an awkward silence in the room. I was seething inside, but I had to remain professional and cool in front of the kids. Aiden felt it, and asked if that A1C number was ok. I told him, "It could be better", and Mr. Wise Guy chimed in, "Yeah. Yes it could." I was already battling enough guilt about failing to bring this number down, and that guilt was compounded by some yahoo who does not live with this disease casting a judgmental tone on me. Because I don't feel bad enough? I later had a talk with his boss.

Return to infancy: Ignorance and Fear

When a child is diagnosed with Type One Diabetes (or any disease, I imagine), one is returned to infancy in more than one metaphorical way. First, I felt returned to infancy in my knowledge base about this disease. I was ahead of the game and knew a little bit because of my education and experience, but I did not know what I did not know. I am sure my husband felt even more behind. Like an infant or toddler, I had to explore my world to learn as much as possible. It is learning that never ceases. I pity those who have zero knowledge about Type One Diabetes and are blind-sided by this diagnosis.

I have read any book that sounded helpful I could get my hands on. Particularly helpful are *Think Like a Pancreas* by Gary Scheiner, *Kids First, Diabetes Second* by Leighanne Calentine, and *Growing Up With Diabetes: What Children Want Their Parents to Know* by Alicia McAuliffe. I combed the JDRF site for as much information as possible. I have learned by trial and error, just like a baby learning his or her new world. I have fallen, succeeded and had my hand slapped in the process.

As a parent, I feel, in a lot of ways, I've been catapulted back to an infancy stage in child care. Talk to any D-mom, and they will tell you they are a walking zombie. It is like having a new baby. You have to feed that baby on a fairly routine schedule. Your sleep is interrupted by mid-night glucose checks, like mid-night feedings in an infant, sometimes more than once per night. The first time your baby slept too long or through the night, I think every mother startled awake and sprang to their baby's bedside to check if they were still breathing. **That heart-stopping fear is back.** If my boys sleep late, I wake up with a start, jump out of bed, and run to their bedside. Each time, I just KNOW they are in a coma. I am certain their sugar dropped undetected. I have to rub their heads, make sure they are responsive, then tell them they can go back to sleep. Or, I check their sugar just to be sure. It is nearly impossible to fall back asleep after being scared to your core.

On our June 2013 family vacation to the beach, I still got up to check the boys in the middle of the night. Towards the end of the trip, I checked the boys in the middle of the night and they were good. Then, they slept late. When I awoke and realized the time, I sprang out of bed and checked on them. Aiden lay flat on his back with arms splayed away from his body. His breathing was shallow and his eyes were half open. Frankly, he looked unconscious or dead. I called his name and he did not respond. I called louder and he still failed to respond. Typically, touching them and asking them if they are ok is enough to elicit a response. If they can respond, then we know they are conscious and alive. When I touched him, he did not respond. My panic level rose with each attempt to rouse him. My thoughts raced. I wanted to scream for Jerry, holler at someone to bring the Diabetes supplies, scream for Glucagon, and yell for 9-1-1 all at once! This all happened in a matter of seconds, but it felt like an eternity. I looked at him and could not believe this was happening! Finally, I grabbed him, shook him, and very loudly called his name. He groaned at me and said, "I'm fine!" Clutching my chest, I stumbled back to my room and attempted to catch my breath. The fear of an unexpected untreated low glucose that causes "dead in bed" is a paralyzing, sleep-depriving fear.

Our routine is to check the boys at their bedtime (around 8pm), and then we check them again sometime before we go to bed (9:30 to 11:30pm). Depending on the glucose level, I get up again. If it is low, I need to treat and recheck. I have to stay up despite overwhelming fatigue to make sure their glucose level is above 100 before I can go to sleep. If it is high, I have to give extra insulin, and then I worry it will go too low. So, I can no longer go to bed early, unless I know my husband will stay up to check on them. Or, I have to set an alarm. And, whichever of us is handling the late check, the other is often awake waiting to hear the result so we can again rest peacefully. I thought my days of "midnight feedings" were over, but now I feed them in the middle of the night at time. I do not think I will rest again until they move out. And, I may not even rest then.

Once all my children were potty-trained, I no longer had to carry a diaper bag with me. I did so for something like four years straight. Now, we are back to having to carry a bag wherever we go. No, there are not diapers in there, but the concept is the same. Keep a "D-Bag" packed and ready to go. The Diabetes bag is packed with emergency Glucagon, hypoglycemia provisions, spare supplies and their meter kits. Like a diaper bag, it goes anywhere the boys go. I know many Mommies who kept a spare diaper in their purse or car when they had babies. Back to infancy, I keep glucose supplies in every car, my purse, and their school book packs

Recently, I took a school field trip with my older non-T1D son, Jace, to Austin, TX, 3 hours away from home. (Yes, now we categorize our children as T1 or non-T1). As I traveled further down the road on a chartered bus, I began to feel more and more helpless and vulnerable. This is what happens! This is what a T1D Mom goes through. My boys have a great age-appropriate understanding of their disease. We have a fabulous REGISTERED NURSE school nurse who really cares about my boys. My husband is fantastic with them.

But, as we got further away from home, my anxiety level increased. On any given day, I am within a few minutes from the school or a cell phone call away to respond to any type of emergency or any of their needs. WHAT if my babies needed me? WHAT if there was an emergency? It has not happened yet, but Murphy's Law would dictate it happen on the day I am hundreds of miles away with no means to hurry back if needed. I felt vulnerable and out of control. I tried and tried, but I could not fight it off. Big giant crocodile tears just started falling. Drop. Drop. Drop. I texted my husband just to vent how I was feeling. He was reassuring, of course, but the tears continued to fall. Simply typing the message to him made me cry. Feeling so vulnerable stinks!

I felt like a crazy woman. I did not want Jace to see me crying. This was HIS Mommy-time. I did not want any of the other adults to see my tears. If I had to explain, it may sound foolish, and it would make me cry harder. I had to dab my eyes, take a deep breath, and divert my thoughts away from this. This is my life now. Too afraid to venture too far unless I know they are in caring and capable hands. Scared to death something will happen to them. Frightened they will need their Mommy and she will not be accessible. I did not exhale until my husband told me he was home. Then, I knew it was all ok.

Every day is new and different. We have our routines of behavior and patterns of testing, but the results are always different. It is the same with the emotions. One day, "I got this". The next, I feel completely inadequate. Befuddled. Confused. Happy. Sad. Angry. Resentful. I still cry. However, when those giant blue eyes and dimpled smiles hug me and insist on extra kisses before I leave or before they go to sleep, it makes this roller coaster ride smoother.

Depression

Overall in life, I try to see the bright side of things. I try not to let things bring me down. Diabetes is a big powerful beast, and it has knocked this Mommy to her knees at times. I have days where all I want to do is go back to bed. Sometimes I do, but usually I cannot because there is too much to do. The Zombie-Mommy needs to catch some extra Zzzs. There are days when the sadness is overwhelming. I am a "fix-it and move-on" kind of gal, and Mommy cannot fix this. I can manage it. I can be a poor substitute as a pancreas, but nothing I do will fix this. That is a tough pill to swallow.

Around the time of Aiden's one-year Diaversary, I was doing my weekly grocery shopping. I have a list to help me, but I think about diabetes constantly every grocery trip. What would be good meals to fix this week? How will that meal affect their blood sugars? How much insulin will I need to give? Every box I pick up, I read the label to see the carb count, then I again think how it would impact them. Or, I see if there are enough carbs, packaged simply, to treat a hypoglycemia episode or be a good pre-PE class snack. As I shopped, these thoughts consumed seemingly every step I took. I grew angry and frustrated. I staved off tears at least three times. I really did not want to look like a crazy woman crying in the middle of Wal-Mart with a grocery cart full of groceries. How could I even explain it? What kept me together was my music, my Bon Jovi. I could just return to the tunes and forget for a few more minutes.

Ordinarily, I do not let it bother me, but as this one year D-Day anniversary approaches, it is plaguing my thoughts. All of it. It's depressing. I am reliving in my mind how scared I was one year ago. I am having flashbacks of the heartbreak, anguish, vulnerability, pain. This steady stream of emotions flares up the anger at the entire situation. I am re-processing the emotions so I can carry on with life.

Should I not be able to just take my list, grab what is needed, and move on? Not anymore. Why can it not just be like it used to be when I grabbed what was on my list then check out? Why do I have to **think** about nearly every consumable item? I went home, and one unrelated snarky remark by my husband just made the flood gates open. The tears fell freely. Of course, he felt horrible, not knowing what burden I was carrying and bottling up. He just hugged me and let me cry.

Crippling Worry

Tagged onto the already deep and complex emotions involved with T1D comes a crippling sense of worry. Hard as I try, I worry. What are their blood sugars? Are their bodies being damage microscopically? What is this doing to their psyche? Will this impact their dating and ability to find a mate? Will they ever be able to live alone? Will I be available if they need me? (I have never been so tethered to my phone in all of my life). Will they wake up in the morning?

I do not mind at all caring for my boys. Mothering is the job I signed up for, for better or for worse. However, I do long for the days when I did not know the approximate carbohydrate count of any random item and the days when I could go to sleep when I felt like it without worrying about my sons' blood sugar or safety. I have found ways to soothe the pain and ease the stress as I do not have the option to sink into depression. There is too much to do and I have too many people depending on me to fall prey to darkness. I use humor, fun times with the kids, alone time with my husband, and gym time to get through the negative thoughts. I use involvement to feel like I am doing something about it. I use Bon Jovi as the dope for my soul to get through. I have to put up a strong front for my boys about this disease as ultimately, I will not be the one managing it. I have to instill in them the knowledge, skills, and self-confidence to manage their lives and Diabetes.

Acceptance is a critical part of Diabetes management for the parents and the children. Diabetes cannot be managed effectively until both accept the diagnosis. With my boys, they accepted their diagnosis so much quicker than I did. The parenting experience of Diabetes is as individual for the parent as it is the child, too. Although our children love us, our investment in their lives is deeper and more intertwined than they will ever understand until they have their own children.

In order to be the best pancreas for my boys, I had to confront and process all of my emotions. This diagnosis has haunted and hurt me. This pain is a deep and lasting emotional hurt for a parent that persists long after the child has moved on. This diagnosis has fatigued me and aged me tremendously over the last year. I have bags under my eyes, dark eye circles, a few extra pounds added, and more grays to color. I realize my emotions are normal, and I let the tears flow when needed. In doing so, I have accepted their fate and I am more driven every day to learn, grow, educate and advocate for them so their lives are as happy and normal as possible.

"...Tonight I'll dust myself off
Tonight I'll suck my gut in
I'll face the night and I'll pretend
I got something to believe in"

Something to Believe In – Bon Jovi

Emotional Roller Coaster

The thing about having identical twins is that you have a constant comparison tool. It began gradually...this feeling that one of my twins, Knox, did not feel well but I could not really put my finger on it. You see, Knox would be trying to run around the living room wrestling with his brothers, but a few minutes later he would grab his bear and go lie down on the couch. I would ask if he was ok, and in his sweet toddler voice he would always say simply, "yes." I will never forget going to the beach a few weeks before his diagnosis. One afternoon he was adamant about not going to the beach, screaming and fighting me the whole way across the pier. I yelled at him in frustration because after all, what 2-year-old does not want to go play in the sand? My Mom agreed to take him back to the condo, and as she held him, he sighed in relief. A couple of weeks later, after days of giving Tylenol off and on and wondering what it was that was bothering him, I decided that for peace of mind I needed to take him to the pediatrician. Upon arrival, the pediatrician gave him a good look and assured me he was on track as far as she was concerned, and asked what it was I had brought him in for exactly. I told her, "I am not sure; he just doesn't seem to have much energy." She agreed with me that was definitely not a common concern for parents of toddlers and suggested that we perform a Complete Blood Count (CBC) to make sure Knox was not anemic. During the next few days we while waiting for the blood work results, Knox started showing the classic signs of Type 1. He would ask for a drink of water and drink the entire contents of the sippy cup immediately after my handing it to him. If he did not have access to a drink at all times, he would become very agitated. The diaper situation was out of control as you can imagine. I had to change him every hour practically throughout the day and night. I told my husband, "He has diabetes" to which he replied, "Naa, it's summer time; he's just really thirsty!" I knew he knew I was right. I received the call from the pediatrician on a Friday afternoon confirming my suspicions and was told we needed to immediately check into the ER. I watched numerous doctors and nurses draw his blood and re-draw his blood, amazed that he did not have ketoacidosis. Again, that is the thing about identical twins. Because I had a constant, virtually identical person in my household to compare him to, we had caught the development of the Type 1 diabetes so early that Knox had not become critically ill yet.

The next few days we spent in the hospital getting Knox's blood sugar under control and learning how to care for him. I knew nothing about diabetes except those warning signs. I thought our new life would require me to give Knox a shot every day, but I felt certain that the change to our lifestyle would be minimal. As I sat at a long conference table with my husband, family, and other newly diagnosed families, tears started streaming down my face as I realized what a huge and cumbersome task we were facing, caring for our tiny T1. I realized that every time he ate virtually ANYTHING he would need a shot. I realized we could no longer leave him in another person's care. No babysitter, no more romantic vacations away with my husband. These of course were my initial, selfish feelings.

A few hours afterwards the nurses came in to show my husband and me how to calculate the insulin needed and how to give the shots. I felt nauseous as I watched the nurses stick the syringe in my little boy. I felt nauseous as I subsequently watched my husband do each injection, meal after meal, each time telling him, "I will do it next time." It went against everything in my mind and body to stick my baby. I could not wrap my mind around it. In the next 24 hours though, I decided I had to suck it up because this was my son, I was his mommy, and if he had to endure this life then I was going to do my part to help him through it.

You can imagine in the coming months the guilt I felt looking back on the beach incident. My husband and I were devastated about the new reality of our son. We mourned for months, going through periods of "We can rock this" followed by "Why Knox?" I questioned all my earlier decisions. Had this happened because I had put him in daycare at one-year-old and he had contracted RSV? His twin brother after all had not caught RSV and had not developed diabetes. Surely I should have kept the nanny longer and this would not have happened. This was completely my fault, I told myself. Still we tried to remind ourselves frequently that at least we got to keep our child. It could always be worse; it was not terminal.

Four months after diagnosis Knox went on an insulin pump and life got slightly less traumatic. We had previously tried to restrict his snacking in an effort to give him fewer shots. As you can imagine, it is impossible to explain to a two year old why we are suddenly now giving him shots but not his brother, and why he can no longer have teddy grahams as a snack but instead has to have cheese and jello. Still, the pump site does have to be changed every three days, sooner if it stops working. Site changes are not fun. Knox calls them his special pokeys. My son is tough as nails, but I never stop dreading site change days. No matter how many you do, as a parent it never feels natural to stick needles in your child.

Today as I write this it has been almost two years since he has been diagnosed. He runs around now wrestling his brothers and giving them a run for their money! His preschool and my family have learned to administer insulin, and we have one babysitter we can trust. I worry daily about what his life will be like after preschool. Will he be made fun of in school? What will it be like to explain to him why can he not go to a friend's house to play without me? Will he eventually grow resentful of his twin who is not T1? Worse yet, will his twin eventually develop T1 too? Most days we are just thankful for modern technology that allows him to live a mostly "normal" life. However, frequently enough diabetes tries to remind us who is the boss by giving us numerous sleepless nights as we stress about low blood sugars, or extremely high blood sugars that we can't figure out a reason for. We realize our ultimate responsibility is making sure this stupid disease does minimal damage to his body until there is a cure. Parents and caretakers of T1 children never stop thinking of diabetes. We never rest soundly. We never stop hating diabetes. We never stop praying for a cure.

Lindsay Houghton

Mother of Collin, Bridger (non-T1D twin), and Knox (T1D since age 2)

Chapter Six: Fostering Independence

As much as this disease is my cross to bear while my sons are small, ultimately, it is their disease. If I could take this disease away from them, I would put the burden on my shoulders in no time. No band-aid will fix it. So, hard as it is for me, I have had to come to terms with the fact that I cannot fix it, but I can learn as much as possible. I can teach them how to manage their disease. I can get involved to help raise money for research. I can make the best of a crummy and unfair situation. Like Lindsey mentioned, it is my job to make sure this disease does minimal damage to their bodies until they can manage it themselves and/or a cure is found.

From the time of Aiden's diagnosis, we have done whatever we could, baby steps, to foster his independence in managing his disease. When Asa jumped aboard uninvited, we did the same for him. Our first step was to offer him a closed choice about the site of his finger stick and his injection when he was still on Multiple-Daily Injections (MDIs). While doing so, we taught the importance of switching sites and the rationale behind it. When they became more used to the idea, we taught them and introduced them into checking their own blood sugars. We stuck with this for awhile, and it worked well because Murphy's Law would insist one or both would feel low while I was in the restroom or shower. Now, they look at their fingers and they can be heard saying, "Nope, I've already stuck this one today", or "This one's getting a little sore", or "I haven't used you today!" They are also able to change the lancets in the lancing devices, and they set the depth to whatever they are comfortable with.

Simultaneously, we were providing age-appropriate education about complications and why checking glucoses and receiving insulin were so critical. We have chosen not to stress their brains or burden their sensitive hearts with all the possible long-term complications. Instead, we focused our education on the two most important complications for their own safety, Hypergylcemia and Hypoglycemia. Basically, they know that if they go too low, they can pass out, and if they are too high, they can become very ill and go into a coma. Both boys are deathly afraid of each. They are too fearful right now to not comply, but I have been warned this will change with the onset of hormones and the ensuing "invincibility" and rebellion of teenager-hood.

From Aiden's diagnosis forward, we have taught all the boys how to read Nutrition Labels. They first learned to recognize where the Total Carbohydrates were listed, and then we incorporated the Serving Size. They quickly learned to count the carbs and double or triple the count for double or triple the serving size. It is common for us to use measuring cups to measure out a serving or put something on the food scale. The boys know they are not limited, but we have to count it accurately so as to give adequate amounts of insulin. Now, they enjoy scooping their own cereal or measuring their own milk into measuring cups. It has become a game.

Also, Aiden understood very early on that he received a certain amount of insulin per grams of carbohydrates consumed (insulin-to-carb ratio). The little genius said, "So, if I don't eat any carbs, I don't have to have any insulin". Perfectly logical conclusion. However, that lead into the discussion about how he was technically correct, but he cannot do that and survive. On occasion, like a big bacon-and-eggs breakfast, this would be alright; however, carbohydrates are essential for his growth and survival. Asa and Aiden can read labels efficiently and tell you which snacks are "free" and which will need to be covered with insulin. When shopping, they will flip boxes or packages over and tell me if it would be a good hypoglycemia treatment or not.

When Aiden was still on MDIs (multiple daily injections), he became interested in administering his own shots. We would draw up the insulin, but he stalled prior to injecting himself. He was just too scared to do it. We let him practice on an orange. And, he got a kick out of Daddy letting him practice with an empty syringe on his arm. Jabbing Daddy several times was really fun! I deferred to Jerry on this one. I have had enough shots and pain just to give birth to these children. I have had my turn as pin cushion; His turn! We lost steam in this training when Asa was diagnosed as we had to start anew with him. Aiden never mastered the task before we began on Insulin Pump Therapy. From time to time, they will have to receive injections for such things as illness or pump failure, and we can reintroduce the task at that time.

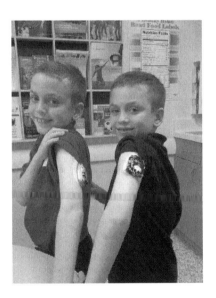

Asa and Aiden, getting their Omnipods (decorated), September 2012

In September of 2012, we started Insulin Pump Therapy for both boys, even though Asa had only been diagnosed one month. That lucky duck did not have to suffer through MDIs for very long! We chose the Omnipod system by Insulet because of its wireless capabilities. We did not want two precious little boys being made fun of at school because they had to carry around a 1990s-pager-looking device attached to their person or some sort of fanny pack to hold supplies. The Omnipod is very concealable on their abdomen, back, upper buttocks, thigh or upper arm. Furthermore, we did not want a device attached to the boys that could easily be damaged on the playground or manipulated by another student. We felt this was the best system for us, although each system has its perks and drawbacks. No matter the system, the control device is profoundly expensive, and we could not bear the thought of having to replace it due to some childhood antics (times two!).

Once we became adjusted to using the Personal Diabetes Manager (PDM) that is the control point of the Omnipod system, we began showing the boys how to use it. First stop was checking their blood sugar on their PDMs. Next, we showed them how to program in the carbohydrates consumed so that the PDM can calculate the amount of insulin needed. If I am over-multi-tasking or not close enough to my son, I will tell him, "Program X amount of carbs into the PDM". They show me for verification and safety, and then they click the button to administer the insulin. (A two-person double-check on insulin is mandatory in the hospital, too!). I feel like being able to do this aids in owning their disease and managing it as well as an eight-year-old can.

Every two to three days the Omnipod site has to be changed. We allow the boys the closed choice of which site to use, and they walk through the process with us by reading the prompts and pushing the programming buttons on the PDM. This served them well later on. Both of our mothers took the Insulin Pump Therapy class with us, but we had only had time to show my mother how to actually do a Pod change prior to our vacation in October (one month after pump therapy began). Our plan was to not burden his mother, Connie, with this task. We had arranged it that their current Pod would last over the visitation time with Jerry's mother every other weekend. We would change it before and after they went to Memaw's. However, I stocked Connie with her own supply of insulin for emergency backup, and I always keep two backup Pods in their Diabetes Kit.

When Jerry and I went out of town for our Anniversary trip weeks after starting on the pump, Aiden's Omnipod failed and alarmed while at Connie's house. (This happens occasionally for different reasons). She was a little frantic about it, and she called my mother to help her. My mother did not receive the call right away. Ever the big helper, Aiden said, "I know what to do, Memaw!" He walked her through an entire Pod change, step by step. He was still only 7-years-old. She was done by the time my mother called her back, and she told us about it later. She was so proud of Aiden. Orientation by fire.

Asa and Aiden are very good with math and well above their grade level in reading. Since Jace is two grades ahead of them, they are learning math concepts above their grade level including multiplication and division. So, we have just begun introducing them into counting their own carbohydrates each meal. I have a dry erase marker board/cork board in the kitchen where I jot down the carb count of what they are currently eating. Jace loves to run over and add up their carbs. Now, the twins add them up, too. Often, I have already calculated and administered their insulin since we try to get the insulin on board as soon as possible (for best effect), but the practice is still good for them.

The next steps are for them to do site changes by themselves and accurately and reliably count carbs and I:C ratios. This may take a year or two for them to learn more advanced math, and they will have to be supervised for awhile for accuracy. Our goal is for them to be able to manage their own meals at school by middle school using the school nurse as a backup or resource person. We are hoping by that age the boys will have demonstrated a level of trust and responsibility that is tied to their understanding and maturity.

Giving them responsibility in their disease management and fostering independence in their diabetes tasks yields responsible independent adults. On a side note, we try to introduce learning as much as possible when they seem receptive. Often though they want to hurry back to their current activity. We have to balance their need for learning with their need to be little boys first.

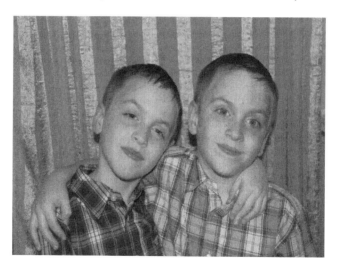

Asa and Aiden on their 8th birthday, October 21, 2012. In this together!

Chapter Seven: Support System

In order to survive any type of trauma, whether it is a death, an illness, or a loss, it is important to develop, seek out, and maintain a strong support system.   Finding and having a reliable support system is critical in dealing with Type One Diabetes, both for the child and the parent(s). What works for one person or family may not be beneficial for all; you have to find what works for you and/or your child.   Good support can come in many forms and it is important to find what works for you while navigating in this new world.   No man is an island, and if you do not have someone or something, Diabetes will incarcerate you.

Family and Friends

As I mentioned before, immediately upon Aiden's diagnosis, I had great support from my immediate family and closest friends. They were ready to listen, eager to learn, and offered support in whatever form they could.   Both sets of our parents were eager to learn and help with the boys. Our moms attended Pump Class with us, and both allow us breaks for dates, overnight visits and/or vacations.   Our older children have admired Aaa and Aiden's strength and bravery in handling their diagnosis and managing their injections and finger pricks.   My friends who do not know or understand refrain from making ignorant remarks. They ask about my boys; they listen when I vent; they take me out so I can forget about being a pancreas for just a little while.

One friend has offered to help and babysit, but our comfort level has not really allowed us to take her up on the offer. There is just too much training involved to keep our boys healthy and safe. Thus, at this time, the only other caretakers we use are our mothers and our daughter. Even then, we worry.

As wonderful as it is, the sympathy and support of family and friends is not nearly as valuable as the input and support from others who have been there or who are walking through the same twisted fairy tale.

Social Networking

Good support comes in many forms, and there may be no better form of support than connecting with others who have been there or walk your walk. Through another friend of mine, I was introduced to Lindsey Houghton who has twins, one of whom has Type One Diabetes. (*So far, only one of her twins has diabetes, and she took it hard when my second twin was diagnosed. It hit a little too close to home for her!*) After Aiden was diagnosed, this mother introduced me to a Facebook group of other Type One Families. This group has provided me with a great sounding board for suggestions, venting and support from others who are walking in my shoes. That type of understanding is priceless. Along with 350+ other people, I use this group as a great resource to share tips, advice, vent, laugh, cry and socialize with others who get it. My friends are fantastic, but they really do not fully get it like another parent of a diabetic child does! I can easily say this group has helped in the acceptance process of the stages of grief. It is great to get the kids together, read about someone else who is experiencing similar things to you, and socialize with other "D-moms". It is great to have someone who speaks your language.

At a recent dinner for our Diabetic parents' group, everyone had their phones out in front of them on the table. We talked and laughed about life and all things Diabetes. A couple of parents answered their ringing phones or texted during the dinner. In a normal situation, this behavior would be viewed as rude. But, each and every one of us at that table understood precisely why those phones were out. Our children with Diabetes were in another's care, and we needed to be accessible to answer questions or respond in an emergency. Meeting such people and attending such events helps parents relate to each other and feel an instant connection with someone who is traveling a similar course as you.

Social Networking

Social networking provides an outstanding opportunity for families looking to connect with others living with Type One Diabetes. The support and comfort it can provide alleviates the need to wait until the next in-person meeting to get help. Being connected with others helps families share personal experiences, knowledge, and encouragement thereby making a positive impact on those living with a life threatening chronic disease such a Type One Diabetes.

Alison Zettle

Creator of Type One Family Network

Mother of Andrew (Diagnosed with T1D at age 6)

I use my personal Facebook to vent, to educate, and to call others to action in fundraising for JDRF. Educating others helps to dispel misconceptions and fears about T1D. Writing has always been therapeutic for me, and I use blogging as an outlet about life in general (marriage, parenting, and now...Diabetes). My blog can be found at www.TwoTooSweet.Com. Getting responses from readers is fulfilling. The comments from other T1D parents helps, and it is gratyifying to think that I am helping another Non-T1D person understand what we experience. I obtain satisfaction in giving another T1D parent a laugh, insight, or help them feel normal.

There are lots of resources online in the Diabetic Online Community (DOC). A newly diagnosed family can seek information and networking through internet searches, support groups, social networking, or resources provided by their local healthcare facility. Feeling isolated, alone, and misunderstood sucks! Find what works for you because you cannot go through this alone. Below are some suggestions:

www.jdrf.org

www.thediabetesoc.com

www.childrenwithdiabetes.com

www.ada.org

Nurturing the Marriage

Any type of trauma can make or break a marriage. Diagnosis of a trying and lifelong disease can tax even the strongest couples. If that which does not kill us makes us stronger, then I should be able to bench press a Hummer by now. I have been so blessed that this has only made my husband and me stronger. We are in this together.

Since we both suffered through failed marriages, we had vowed to ourselves and each other to learn from our past mistakes and not fail again. One thing we have always done is make our marriage a priority. We still go on dates. We go on annual anniversary vacations. We have adult time each evening after the kids' bedtime where we just spend time together talking or watching television. We talk on the phone a couple of times per day. We send little messages to each other and try to do nice things for each other. We respect each other and allow time apart as individuals. We did this before Diabetes invaded our lives, and now it has become even more critical as it allows each of us an escape, the ability to exhale, and recharge our batteries.

Jerry and I have had to deal with more than our fair share of nonsense in our marriage (that's another book or Dr. Phil episode!). Yes, it has caused fights sometimes, but we have learned how to communicate more effectively with each other, and we have emerged stronger as a couple. We have an unwritten rule that we have each other's backs, right or wrong! (If wrong, we'll discuss in private later). These trials have strengthened our resistance, our resolve, and our resilience, so when T1D was thrown onto our plates, we did not turn against each other. Rather, we turned *towards* each other. We shared our feelings, and we held hands and dove into this together. Although this stinks for both of us, I do not think it impacted him as hard emotionally. It's a Mommy thing. Regardless, when I am overwhelmed emotionally, he is there to hold me and reassure me. He allows me to cry, vent, and get away when I need to. It's OUR disease to manage, those are OUR boys.

In managing Diabetes, one parent has to take the driver's seat. It does not matter who, just as long as there is a Pilot and a Co-Pilot. I am the Pilot, and I have a great Co-Pilot. He leaves all the appointments, prescriptions, decisions and adjustments to me. There is no sense in duplicating efforts or tripping over each other. Since healthcare is my bag, and I am home more, I am the Pilot. (He "pilots" all the computers, technology and networking since that is his bag). As a good Co-Pilot should, he is great about managing their care when I am not around, and he tries new things and shares his findings with me, too. Jerry is great about analyzing insurance coverage and prescription coverage so we can find the right plan for us. He attends any appointment he can...and if he cannot go, he is calling before I can check out. It is definitely a team effort, and it works for us.

Diabetes is a tough, demanding and lonely disease, and managing it is easily more than enough work for two people. For us, I guess we have the work of four people. I feel sorry for the single parents whose child/children are diagnosed because I do not know what I would do if I did not have Jerry to help me and to lean on. So, if things are not going well or your partner is not a good Co-Pilot, then expand your support system in other ways. Access the resources of your hospital or clinic. Seek help through your church or through counseling. It is bad enough Diabetes is robbing our children of part of their childhood; do not let it rob you of your marriage.

Involving the Kids

Our local Children's Hospital supports an annual camp specifically for Type One Diabetes patients and their siblings (for a much larger fee, if space allows). There is only one other girl in Asa and Aiden's school who has diabetes, and she is two grades ahead of them. I felt it was important for Aiden to meet other children with

Diabetes, to have something that was just for him, and to have fun. Involvement for the children promotes acceptance, support and confidence. So, in June of 2012, I sent him and Asa to Camp Aurora. It is a medically safe and educationally supportive environment for children with Diabetes of all ages. I chose to send Asa, also, because I felt more comfortable keeping my twins together; I did not want Aiden to be alone. Also, I figured Asa needed the exposure, too, in case he later developed Diabetes. Little did I know it would be so soon afterwards.

At Camp, they had fun playing each day. They learned new sports and games and were challenged. One of the highlights of their camp time was getting to meet a Dallas Mavericks professional basketball player. They also spent time teaching the children more about Diabetes and managing Diabetes while having fun. It was a fun experience for both boys, and they are looking forward to going back in 2013. At least this time we will not have to pay so much for Asa!

There are other camps geared towards Type One Diabetic Children including the Texas Lions Camp and Camp Sweeney. Others have sent their children to these overnight away camps, but I was not ready to do that with Aiden alone at age seven. I explained the overnight camps to him last year. He seemed okay with the idea at first until I told him it was for one or two weeks. Then, he said, "Maybe when I'm twelve, Mommy!" I am not sure why 12 is the magic age, so I plan to keep introducing the idea of these camps to both boys now. I will leave it up to them as to if and when they are ready to be away from home and Mommy that long. When they are ready, I am certain they will handle it much better than I will!

Getting Involved

I have been familiar with JDRF (Juvenile Diabetes Research Foundation) for a long time. If nothing else, I was fascinated by their acronym since it was a combination of my and my husband's initials together (Jerry D & Rhonda Fuselier). We were reintroduced to JDRF in the hospital when Aiden received his Rufus Backpack. I read through every single thing we were given in the hospital, and I continued my education and research on JDRF's website. I also looked extensively at the American Diabetes Association's website, but I prefer JDRF since they are dedicated to Type One.

In the past five years, my daughter and I have run 5Ks recreationally, and I combed JDRF's site hoping they had a benefit 5K. I found instead they had an annual Walk to Cure Diabetes. I researched it and asked my Facebook compadres about their involvement. In July of 2012, I registered our team, Aiden's Army, to participate in the Walk to Cure Diabetes in October 2012. Fundraising and making T-shirts were uncharted territories to me, but I wanted to do what I could to raise money for JDRF to support their efforts in research.

I named our team and designed and ordered our T-shirts prior to Asa's diagnosis. The T-shirt company literally called the day Asa was in the hospital saying our shirts were ready, so there was no renaming the team at that point. Our 2013 will be named *The A2 Team (A-squared)* to incorporate both boys' names. We earned over $2000 for JDRF through our family team in 2012. I did not think that was too bad for a rookie. In the process, I met new people and learned other tricks and methods to raise money. Our goal will be larger for 2013. The Walk is a fun and healthy family activity, and it allows me to feel like I am doing *something* to help find a cure for my boys. If I cannot fix it myself, I can help those who can! Getting involved gives me something to believe in.

Currently, my local JDRF representative and I are trying to get my boys' school district to host an annual Kids Walk to Cure Diabetes. Because they are identical twins and because of Diabetes, my boys are well known in their school. This is a great way to get kids involved in learning about Type One Diabetes and is a fun way to raise money for a cure. In the future, I hope to find a way to host or run a 5K that will benefit JDRF. There are many ways to get involved in the Diabetes community to feel like you are doing something about it and assist in finding a cure.

Getting Involved

My daughter, Kate, was diagnosed at age 7 and, of course, you always think "Why her?", "Why us?" I know why now--to be involved with JDRF, mentoring others, and being a support system in the community of T1 parents and children. We found purpose and meaning in her diagnosis.

I think my strongest calling to be involved is to be mentor and support other parents as they find out their child has been diagnosed. The first family I met after we were diagnosed was another family whose child would be attending our school in the fall. The mother and I sat in my family room and talked for hours, our children played for those hours and to this day we continue to support each other, even though I have moved away. There is a bond that is almost always felt when you meet and talk with someone going through the same thing you are going through. I feel if my child and I can help a new family through this transition, and even develop lasting friendships from it, then I have found a positive outcome of my child having Type 1 Diabetes.

My other "involvement" passion is JDRF's Walk to Cure Diabetes. A friend came to me after my child was diagnosed and asked me if it was okay to have a walk at our school to raise money for JDRF in honor of my child. Of course, I said "yes!" with tears in my eyes. Our school walk was great success and through it I learned more about a BIG walk that JDRF hosted every year. So I decided we needed a team that would walk with us and support our family and most importantly our child. That first year I did not put a lot of effort into raising the money, it was more about raising awareness and the support. We had about 60 walkers and even raised a nice amount of money. Since then we have had a team every year, and each year our donations to find a cure has increased, which is a nice bonus. The support that comes out of our team each year is what is amazing! The love that surrounds our child makes my heart happy and makes me want to do this walk every year until we find a cure.

Amy Feighner (Team Captain of Kate's Carb Counters)

Top Family Team Earner for JDRF Walk to Cure Diabetes (Fort Worth) in 2012

Chapter Eight: Better Left Unsaid

When your child is diagnosed with Type One Diabetes (or any disease), people often try to soothe the parent or cast blame and judgment. Way too many people are horribly misguided and misinformed about Diabetes and they immediately think Type One and Type Two are similar or one-in-the-same. The only similarity is in the name and the organ it affects. In a perfect world, the two diseases would have different names to distinguish them from each other. I have been blessed with good support from family, friends and co-workers, but I still hear the occasional stupid, ignorant, or offensive remark. Other Type One Parents have shared things they have heard and experienced, too, and I never cease to be amazed at the ignorance and insensitivity of others. Granted, I think most people mean well, but they do not stop and think before saying things that are better left unsaid.   It is best to expect strange comments from people and remember that before diagnosis, I did not know very much about T1D either (but perhaps I was wise enough to keep comments to myself). If you expect it, then it does not sting quite as badly and you can be prepared to respond.

When a child is diagnosed with Juvenile Diabetes, a parent is suddenly bombarded with an over-abundant amount of information, has to adjust to a different lifestyle and disease management, and is often sleep-deprived, confused, depressed, and overwhelmed. The entire family is impacted. To boot, well-meaning friends, extended family, and sometimes strangers say the damndest things to a parent who is trying to cope with keeping their baby **alive** and healthy (and some of us, more than ONE child!).

Functioning as a pancreas is a full-time job; functioning as more than one is overtime! We understand people mean well, but honestly, some of the ignorant remarks can be hurtful. It is like adding insult to injury. We understand not everyone fully understands this disease, as we all did not understand either until it was thrown forcefully into our laps. Now, we try to educate so we can improve understanding and perhaps inspire another person to donate time or money to finding a cure. However, if it has been a rough night, or the person has a particularly indignant or judgmental tone, or the person says something horrifying in earshot of our innocent babies, it is really hard to bite our tongues! If you do not know what to say, do not say anything …. except, "I'm sorry" or "I'll be thinking about you" or "How can I help?"

With great reminders from awesome fellow Type One Parents from our cool forum, I will let you read some of the wonderful, well-meaning things that have been said to some or all of us. In no particular order:

1. *"It's just diabetes; he'll be fine!"* Yes, yes, *it could be worse*, but please do not undermine the seriousness and gravity of this disease. It is a constant and every day struggle to manage and keep your child alive and healthy. And, NO, you do not have a crystal ball to tell us how our boys will turn out! Frankly, this statement is dismissive of a mom or dad's mourning of their child's pre-diabetic life and the "perfectness" and innocence of their childhood. It's dismissive of a mom or dad's effort and energy spent into managing an often unruly disease!

2. *"It'll make you a better mother"* What the…? Did I SUCK before so I needed a life-altering diagnosis to get me to fly right? Having your child diagnosed with T1D **WILL** require you to be more diligent, organized and overseeing about

certain aspects of your child's life and medical care(until he or she can manage his/her disease on his/her own), but it will not change your basic parenting. Diabetes will not prevent your child from sitting on the therapist's couch because of your newfound parenting prowess!

3. *"All he has to do is take insulin."* Yes, he has to take insulin. But, it is not so simple. We have to check blood sugars via finger-stick AT LEAST four times per day (but up to 10 times per day if needed). *Did you read that? Four to ten times per day* we have to inflict pain and cause our babies to bleed! We have to count every carbohydrate he eats. We have to become math geniuses and administer a set dose of insulin based on the blood sugar and the amount of carbohydrates consumed. What works well one day, will fail miserably the next. Managing Diabetes is a fantastic mix of science, math, voodoo and sorcery to get that perfect unattainable "normal" blood sugar or Hemoglogin A1C level! We have to worry about highs, lows, complications, Endocrinology appointments, Ophthalmology appointments, Pediatric appointments, quarterly venipunctures for lab work, and middle of the night blood sugar checks. So, yes, insulin is the primary medication that maintains his life, but that is not "all"!

4. *"You can't have diabetes, you're too thin!"* Again, T1D is NOT a lifestyle disease. T1D an autoimmune disorder wherein the pancreas is attacked and can no longer produce its own insulin. At the onset of the disease, the patient is essentially starving to death because glucose cannot enter into the cells (because insulin carries it into the cells), so most often, the patients ARE very thin. So, thanks for noticing! (Just for the record, I DO wish someone would say that to me when looking at my fabulous post-five-babies abs

or my caboose!) On the flip side, it would be equally inappropriate to say, "You must have Type 2 Diabetes because you're such a cow!"

5. *"You shouldn't have given him/her too much soda (or other sugary substance) because it causes diabetes"*. To try to explain the difference between Type One and Type Two Diabetes can be taxing. Some people just want to be "right" and are indignant if educated. Our children did NOT develop diabetes because of too much sugar. He did not overdose on jelly doughnuts! Saying T1D was "caused" by sugar is like saying your baby's hair color was caused by the prenatal vitamins you took. Unrelated. Genetics aided in both their hair color and their propensity to develop an autoimmune disorder. They developed diabetes because these wicked little antibodies decided to have a war inside their tiny bodies, and the pancreas was killed by this "friendly fire". Poor diet, nutrition, and lifestyle CAN lead to **Type 2** Diabetes because the person is taxing the limits of the pancreas's capabilities (and other organs). It was nothing I fed my child; had nothing to do with my pregnancy; had nothing to do with my career choice. My boys did not get diabetes because I let them eat too much candy or play too many video games. Trust me, we did not cause this disease by poor parenting and indulgence, and we'd do anything in the world to take it away from our babies!

6. *"I know how you feel; My cat has diabetes"* I know people love their pets (I adore my worthless dogs), and there may be some people who love their pets more than they love their kids. However, for most of us, our kids are our **top** priority! So, I am sorry you have to limit Garfield's lasagna and give him a shot in the scruff of his neck twice a day (and hope he doesn't scratch or bite you), but it is NO

comparison to the illness of a child! As a matter of fact, I told my veterinarian that my dogs are just going to have to be dogs because I have CHILDREN to pay for and medicate. The dogs fall to the bottom of the priority list in that regard! Please do not compare your animal to my human sons! Furball's Diabetes is just as different from a human's Diabetes as is his ability to lick himself.

7. *"You STILL have to poke his finger?"* Unfortunately, when we all went to Diabetes Education classes, we did NOT walk away with mental telepathy. We cannot guess what a blood sugar is at any given moment, and it can change dramatically in minutes. So, even those who wear Continuous Glucose Monitors STILL have to check their sugars because the CGM is only a tool. Until new devices are developed or a cure is found, we have to check blood sugars 4-10 times per day. By adulthood, the tips of their fingers will be as hardened as a spinster's heart!

8. *"That's good! He has a pump, so now you can control it!"* Regardless of the method of insulin delivery, Diabetes is a disease that controls us. The only thing the pump changes is that the child does not have to get a shot every time he/she needs insulin. Insulin delivery options are a personal choice, and Diabetes can be managed on Multiple Daily Injections (MDIs) just as well as with a pump.

9. *"Cinnamon. Honey. Alkaline Diet. The Root of Some Exotic Plant"* *Holy crap, really!?* WHY didn't someone tell my Endocrinologist about this? Man, we are wasting so much money on supplies and insulin, research and treatments when the simple solution has been sitting on the spice rack all along? I will repeat: There are a lot of books out there about Diabetes cures and treatments. Most of these refer to Type 2 Diabetes and will NOT help my sons. (They may or may not help a Type 2 Diabetic either). Trust me, if it would,

I would have tried it already….multiple times. Unfortunately for them, none of that will take away the attack on their tiny pancreases. I wish it would.

10. **"When will she grow out of it?"** This disease is not like tennis shoes, new dresses, middle school boyfriends, or colic! They do not outgrow it. (Don't we all WISH this was temporary?!) Junior and the Big D better get cozy and friendly, because until a cure is found, they will live with this disease for the rest of their lives. *crossing fingers* Maybe one day…

11. **"What was his/her diet like before diabetes? How much did you have to change?"** Beating a dead horse here, but bad dietary choices did not cause this disease. Saying diet caused my identical twin sons' diabetes is like saying Rock 'n' Roll caused Elvis. Personally, we changed almost nothing in my house. I already cooked lean meats, vegetables, fruits, low fat dairy. Chips, cookies, and fast food are the exceptions in my house, not the rule. Sugar was dramatically limited. The only change we had to make was to suddenly become a food diary and look-up and memorize the carbohydrate counts on tons of different foods. Putting this information into my database has caused other things to be tossed into the Recycle Bin in my head. I do not know what the year model of my car is or what year I was born, but I can tell you that one hushpuppy averages 8 carbohydrates each, and the average banana is 30 carbs!

12. **"You don't have the diabetes under control YET?"** We do not control Diabetes, it controls us. Diabetes is the Honey Badger….it just does not care! It is like putting the reins on an untamed horse. Sometimes, pulling on the reins will work, sometimes the horse will buck the other way. As parents, because we love our children, we try everything to

keep Diabetes under control (see # 3 above). The only control we have is consistency, timing and SWAG'ing!

13. **"I guess he/she should just have a salad. I guess he/she shouldn't eat the bread"** These are things we have heard when asking a waiter/waitress if they happen to have the Nutrition Facts of their entrees or meals. Because people look at you like you are bat-crap crazy when asking, we feel the need to explain that our child has T1D, and we just want the carbohydrate counts of the over-priced foods we are purchasing from your establishment so we can appropriately dose the insulin. We are not food critics or the Health Department; we are loving concerned parents who want to dose our children correctly. Relax! Instead of "No, we don't have it available" or *"I'm sorry"*, we get Diabetes management advice from a waitperson who makes $2.15/hr. I guess having a name tag that says both "Texas Roadhouse" and "Suzie" on the same piece of cheap plastic makes you an Endocrinologist and a Nutritionist! Skip college, get the plastic tag!

14. **"That's what sitting home eating potato chips will do for 'ya!"** If this had been me, I think I would be facing an assault and battery charge right now.

15. **"Type One. That's the good (or bad) kind, right?"** I did not know that any disease was good, especially in an innocent child who did nothing to deserve this! Diabetes is difficult and life-altering, not good.

16. **"Why do you poke her finger so much?"** Says fatty-fatty-two-by-four Grandpa who is consuming two desserts after a meal with over 2000 calories while injecting 320 units of insulin in one sitting (trust me, this is an enormous amount of insulin). All the while, his foot is falling off, he is going blind, and his penis quit working years ago because his

Diabetes is out of control. **Why, you ask**? Because, she has T1D; I love her; I care about her health; Things can change in an instant; and, I don't want her to be in your condition by the time she is 40. *(I don't think she'll have to worry about her penis, but I digress! You get the point!)* Are those enough reasons to check more than two times per day?

17. **"It's JUST Juvenile Diabetes!"** Why yes, yes it is. Thanks for pointing that out! I had not noticed! Sheesh, really? Because when they hit 18, it is still freaking Diabetes, they just are not juveniles anymore. They will not outgrow it! They will live with this craptastic disease until the day they die, and as parents, we hope our hard work will mean they do not die sooner than the next brat!

18. **"Oh, they get used to it!"** Who really gets used to being stabbed with a needle several times per day or pricking their finger before every meal? The child may stop crying or complaining because it is become part of their routine (or they know it is a necessary evil), but I do not think anyone ever gets used to it. People get acclimate to subpar conditions on a routine basis. Abuse, hunger, chronic pain, neglect, and corruption. (Babies in orphanages quit crying for food when they realize their cries go unanswered. Doesn't mean they're not still hungry.) I am not sure how that is reassuring. The physical pain of this disease becomes an unfortunate part of life.

Some days, it is easy to ignore or overlook insensitive remarks. Other days, it is a labor of love to not say what you would really like to say. I try to take the high road and use these incidents as an opportunity for education about Type One Diabetes. Perhaps, if one person understands better, then they will not repeat their mistake, and they may be compelled to become involved.

Chapter Nine: Boys Will Be Boys

It's easy to get caught up focusing primarily on Diabetes. Diabetes is an important part of my boys' lives, but is not the focus of their lives. As a Mommy, I am so afraid of the immediate and long-term problems associated with T1D. Yet, despite the disease, we have to remember that there are still two little boys inside - little boys who still need to experience a childhood. It saddens me they have to deal with this craptastic disease, so I focus on making sure they are not denied the chance to be a kid as much as is plausible. As parents, it is our job to parent them, prepare them for adulthood, *and* act as their substitute pancreas. As children, it is Asa and Aiden's job to learn, grow, play, and be little boys!

Normalcy

First, I have made sure my friends and the boys' friends know that it is acceptable to still invite my boys to birthday parties. As have other diabetic parents have, I have encountered people fearful to invite because they think the diabetic child would not be allowed to have the available treats, or they feel like they must provide a sugar-free snack. As I have told them, please still invite them. Prepare or offer nothing different than you ordinarily would. You be the hostess, I will be the pancreas. I do not want them to miss out on any celebrations because of Diabetes.

Second, it takes more diligence and planning, but I have made it a point to carry on with summer time activities, outings, and vacations as we did before Diabetes plopped his big butt in our lives. I pack a bag with a few juice boxes and snacks to go in with their kits. Over the summer, we went to the beach. Diabetes tagged along. That involved a tremendous amount of planning on my part...planning my boys never knew anything about. All they knew was they were going on vacation. Basically, on top of packing for the entire family, I packed an extra bag for Diabetes with an abundance of supplies. I packed a cooler with drinks and snacks and insulin.

Each summer, I like to take my boys to local recreational places. Even though I like to be early and the first one in everywhere I go, I have altered my way of thinking and my habits. I have found it a bit simpler to go right after lunch. I will feed and dose the boys for an early lunch, then pack the same D-bag with kits and snacks. This alleviates the stress of trying to find an appropriate lunch at the right time, and it alleviates the excess cost of feeding five or more children while out. The boys still get to go to the museum, trampoline park, swimming, and/or the zoo. They get to be kids; I get to be the organizer and pancreas.

A child with Diabetes can do most anything as long as he or she allows for Diabetes in his or her schedule. Diabetes is a petulant child and will tolerate nothing less.

Kids First

Recently, my mom told me how it drove her crazy when the twins left their meter kits messy after checking their sugars. I insist they throw their trash away, but sometimes they forget. However, they are bad about checking their sugars and not placing their supplies neatly back under the elastic bands in the meter kit. I framed it for her like this: They are still two little boys who have to deal with a very adult illness. Fifteen minutes or so before every meal, they have to *stop* being little boys and come cause themselves to bleed and receive insulin. Too often, they have to stop playing to treat an out-of-normal-range glucose level. Most other children do not have to deal with such a burdensome task. So, if they hurry and make a hasty exit to run back and continue playing, that is alright with me. I will play the role of tidier and pancreas while they perform their little boy jobs!

As I mentioned before, fostering the boys' independence in managing their Diabetes is an added task of our parenting. This has to be coupled with still allowing them to be kids. Whenever possible, we do not want them treated any differently than any other classmate. For example, Asa became very upset at school in second grade because everyone received two birthday cupcakes, but he had only received one. He had already gone to the nurse, checked his blood sugar and been dosed with insulin for one cupcake. The teacher and school nurse were reluctant to allow him more, and he was heart-broken. He came home very angry at the injustice of it all. At that point, I told her that if a similar situation occurs in the future, she can just tell him or the teacher what the carb count is on the extra treat, and he can program the PDM himself. Win, win! He is a kid first, Diabetes second.

Discipline and Expectations

We attempt to deal with Diabetes in a healthy way so as not to be enslaved by it. We disallow any sort of pity party, or Diabetes will move in completely and dominate our lives. I think it would be easy to fall into the trap of pitying a child for having an illness. On some level, I do pity them, and I'd take this from them double time if it meant they never had to poke their fingers again. Unfortunately, that is not going to happen. Jerry and I are still molding two little boys hopefully into healthy productive adult members of society. Preparing them for adulthood is our primary job. Pitying them and letting them get away with murder because we feel sorry for them is doing them a disservice. Instead of adults with Diabetes, they would be adult jerks with Diabetes. Asa and Aiden still have chores. They still have expectations for their behavior. They have to do their homework. They clean their room. They are rewarded and praised, and they are disciplined when necessary.

With that being said, we do have to take into consideration what their glucose level is with their behavior. Sadly, high and low blood sugars can yield very ugly attitudes and bad behaviors. That is not their fault. As I have told family members, teachers, and friends, if Asa and Aiden are acting out, especially if it is out of character, then check their sugar. If it is normal, then they are really going to get it! If it is wicked high or low, then we deal with that first and the behavior next. They are still held accountable for their actions, but if you know their sugar is off, you know it is not entirely their fault and you can wave some things off. Aiden especially, as he did before diagnosis, is very prone to behavioral disturbances if his glucose level is too high. Not always, but he can become angry and combative at times. There have been plenty of occasions where I have had to take a deep breath, not take it personally, and isolate him until his sugar is improved. When the glucose level is normalized, I get my sweet boy back. Exhale, and cut them a little slack when Diabetes is the culprit.

In the end, however, we refuse to allow our boys to use Diabetes as a scapegoat, a crutch, or an excuse. Although some provisions have to be made to make room for Diabetes, our expectations have not changed. Our boys are expected to do their best at school, behave well, be good citizens, and play nicely with others. Currently, both boys make straight A's and have received good conduct awards.

Dress It Up and Make It Fun

Finally, Diabetes may not like wearing a dress, but we try to dress it up and make it as fun as possible. Frankly, it sucks, but we have to find light where we can. I have purchased tons of decorated duct tape to put over their Omnipods so they have some flare and personality to them. SpongeBob, Camouflage, Batman, Spiderman...we have them all. Second, following suggestions from other D-parents, I have made cool sleeves or we buy cool wraps to put over the Omnipod sites. This helps secure and protect the site (since it's supposed to last three days), and it gives the boys something cool to wear. They enjoy picking out the designs or colors on the Vet Wrap we use over their pods. Finally, it would be monotonous and boring if every hypoglycemic episode was treated with juice. To make it more fun, we use pre-packed candies to treat low blood sugars. If they have to have this crummy disease and experience scary hypoglycemia, then at least we can treat it in a fun way.

Asa and Aiden have Diabetes, but there is so much more to them. Diabetes is a blemish in my boys' childhoods. Besides keeping them healthy and avoiding complications, my goal is to make sure they experience a happy and relatively normal childhood. They play. They fight. They go on field trips. They ride bikes and go to the park. They play video games and read. They participate in after school clubs. And, they were even able to attend a Bon Jovi concert with Mommy. With a little planning and foresight, I can keep Diabetes from ruining their fun, and let them be boys!

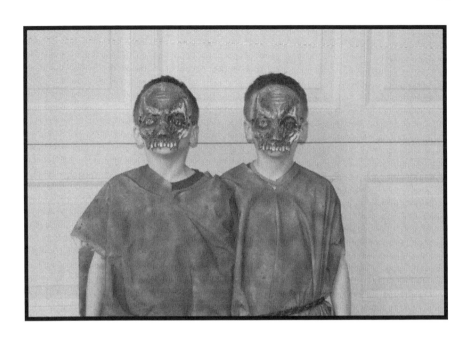

Asa and Aiden still get to do things, like trick-or-treat!

Two-Headed Monster, October 2012

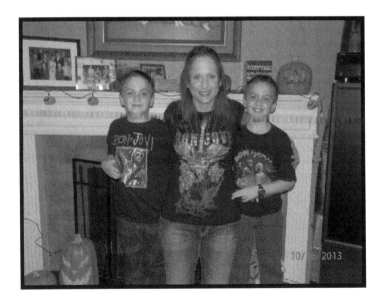

Going to see Bon Jovi with Mommy, Oct 2013

Chapter Ten: Colossal Failures

Diabetes does not care how old you are, what color you are, where you live, or what your education level is. It does not care if you stay-at-home or work full-time outside the home. It cares about nothing, and despite our best efforts to manage this beast, it still punches through and shows us who is in charge! Despite our diligence and best efforts, we have had some colossal failures in our attempts to manage Diabetes. The guilt a D-Mom carries around has no boundaries, and causing such "failures" makes the angst grow larger. When I do not get it right, my boys are the ones who suffer. My guilt is temporary; their consequences are real, tangible and threatening. These are not our finest moments, but we will tell the tales so that others can learn, laugh, and realize its ok to screw up now and then. You are not alone. Some days are great, some are good, and some are terrible. Tomorrow is a new day.

Missed or Miscalculated Boluses

To begin with, we dosed our boys' insulin during or towards the end of their meal. Ideally, it is best to dose before a meal so that the insulin is working by the time the carbohydrates are processed into glucose in the bloodstream. However, pre-meal dosing is difficult in young children because they may or may not finish their meal and/or they may want more. Since we had to wait and see what the boys had actually consumed, sometimes we walked away and did something else while they are eating. Most of the time, they call out, "I'm done; I'm ready for my insulin!" However, if more pressing issues are at stake, like who is going to get back to the Xbox or TV program the quickest, they may forget. If we are doing other things, we may forget, too. (We have since progressed to pre-dosing based on a predicted amount of carbs to be consumed since they are now older children, and we add extra insulin via pump if needed).

My husband handled the breakfast one day, and I handled lunch. Aiden's pre-lunch glucose was 425! His pump site was fine, and he felt ok. So, I asked Jerry, "What did Aiden have for breakfast?" I wondered if Aiden had eaten more than he told his Daddy or Daddy has miscalculated. Also, I wondered *what* he ate because if it impacted him this negatively, we need to avoid that meal in the future! Jerry started to answer me when he stopped mid-sentence! "Crap, I forgot to bolus him!" Oops! So, I gave Aiden correction insulin and insulin for his lunch. Live and learn. Immediately after lunch, we went shopping. 30-45 minutes into shopping, we had to stop and check Aiden's sugar because he felt low. So, on the sidewalk outside of Kohl's, I checked and discovered a glucose level of 45! 425 to 45 in just over an hour!

Lessons Learned: Diabetes is boss, men cannot multi-task, and apparently, shopping causes hypoglycemia.

Shortly after Courtney's wedding in June of 2012, the boys and I traveled to her town to visit and have lunch. We ate at a Mexican restaurant for lunch. Aiden ate his birth weight in chips and salsa (as he usually does). I calculated a ball-park estimate of the amount of chips he ate. I figured up the approximate carb count for his kids' meal. We treated ourselves to sopapillas, and I looked that up, too. What I could not find was the carb count for honey. Aiden lathered his sopapilla in honey. It took a SWAG (Scientific Wild-Ass Guess) at the carbs. Once I had calculated it all, I gave Aiden the LARGEST single bolus dose of insulin he ever had thus far in his life! He was scared and I was equally nervous. I KNEW he would drop low on our way home.

Apparently, my SWAG was crap. Adding insult to injury and complicating the issue, Aiden added more honey to his sopapilla after I had dosed him. Four or five hours later, I went out to dinner with my girlfriends. Jerry checked Aiden's sugar before dinner. Drum roll, please…..454! Yep, OVER 400 despite his largest dose of insulin to date! I immediately felt AWFUL and embarrassed. I am supposed to be the Pilot and I just rolled the airplane! In his ever sympathetic way, Jerry reassured me, "It's ok. I'll glue his foot back on later!"

Lesson learned: Diabetes is in charge and honey has 17g carbs per tablespoon! (Since we were still new then, we have since learned that big meals like this cause the boys to spike 4 to 6 hours after the meal due to the high fat and protein content.)

Finally, in January, JDRF had an awards dinner for all teams who raised money during the October 2012 Walk to Cure Diabetes. My mom and I took the twins to the dinner. Now, a logical person would think there would be carb counts available or pre-calculated at a DIABETIC dinner, but there was not *(that suggestion will be made for next year!).* We enjoyed a catered Texas Barbecue dinner. Again, I calculated much of the dinner with SWAG'ing. Some carb counts I knew by heart, others were guesses. Each boy was given insulin ASAP! Using the pump makes it easier to allow for adding insulin doses for seconds, dessert, etc, and this is what we did. Each boy had a piece of pecan pie for dessert, and I estimated 40g carb per piece. Since we were celebrating and this was a RARE treat, they were allowed a second piece. 40g and dosed for all of it.

On the way out, we stopped at a candy shop, and the boys got a small sucker that was 15g carbs. With more insulin added, they ate the lollipop on the way home. Now, given all the sugar, I figured they would be high before bed since it was getting close to bedtime and the insulin did not have time to fully act. After showers, we checked their blood sugars. Asa was high, but not too bad. In the low 200s I think. Aiden, 550! We repeated, 549! FIVE HUNDRED? Aiden is super-sensitive to carbs, but this was crazy!

Ever the sensitive one, Asa started freaking out and bombarding me with questions. *"What number makes you go into a coma, Mommy!? I don't want Aiden to go into a coma! You need to take him to the hospital now!"* It is difficult to try to correct a situation when you have to calm down a panicking child! *"ASA! Mommy's got this! Aiden's going to be okay!"* The joke was on me. Clearly I had dropped the ball and had nothing. Ever the genius, my husband asked, *"Did you give him insulin?!"* *"Um, YES, and LOTS of it!"* (Thanks for stating the obvious!) Apparently, not enough though. I gave Aiden correction insulin. I gave him a big glass of water. I reassured both boys I would come up and check them in one hour. Asa begged, *"Will you check him at 9:30, Mommy?!"* (That was 45 minutes away). Ok. I agreed to whatever to get him to settle down! They went to bed. Aiden was otherwise fine.

The anxiety consumed Asa and he started freaking Aiden out. They got out of bed at 9 pm and asked to recheck Aiden. Ok, whatever. This time, "HIGH" is all it said (I lied and told them it was the same lest I induce more panic in either boy). His sugar was climbing and off the charts! Yikes! I had to recheck every two to three hours during the night and give correction insulin. By morning, it was in the 200s, and he normalized out over the course of the day. I was exhausted.

A few weeks later, I saw a pecan pie for sale at Wal-Mart. Curious, I looked at the nutrition facts. On this small 8-inch pie, one piece was 77g carbs. Uh oh. The Pilot nose-dived this time! That means that JDRF pecan pie was at least 100g per slice. Bad SWAG. Bad. I miserably under-dosed my carb-sensitive child for that pie.

Lessons Learned: Diabetes is a rebellious teenager, I suck at SWAG, and I hope Jerry gets really good at his glue work!

Who's on First?

As I mentioned, our boys are identical twins. During the day, we can tell them apart. We usually do so by asking, "What's your name?" but we have other methods, too. Clothes, shoes, scars. Our twins share a room. One bed is preferred, so they have compromised and switch beds weekly. To further compound the issue, they crawl in bed with each other about half the time, too! Needless to say, checking blood sugars in the middle of the night requires due diligence. Despite our best efforts, we still both screw it up now and then. Who's in what bed? Which meter is whose? Who's on first?

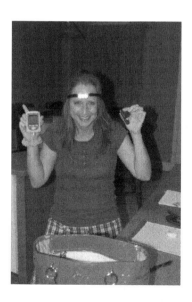

My Spelunker attire to sneak in and check blood sugars after bedtime

More than once, I have examined the designated child, determined him to be Twin A or Twin B and checked the glucose. After seeing the result, I realize I have switched boys. Not too big a deal as long as I document the correct sugar on the correct boy's clipboard. Not too big a deal as long as we're not dealing with correcting a high or low blood sugar.

One night when I was working, Jerry adopted my Spelunker look and checked the boys before retiring for the night. He checked "Asa" and he was normal. He checked "Aiden", and he was high and needed correction. He set "Aiden's" pump to administer correction bolus. It kept giving the error message "PDM communication error. Out of range". He moved the PDM closer. He turned it around. He laid it on his body. Nothing fixed the error. At that point, he realized it was out of range because he was holding the wrong PDM up to the wrong boy, which means the PDM was trying to give insulin to Asa when Aiden needed it. Try as he may, Jerry could not get the correction insulin to cancel. He was afraid to cross the room, let the PDM get in range, and give insulin to the child who did not need it. (Now we know we can hit cancel as soon as the insulin starts).

So much for letting the boys sleep. He finally had to deactivate the pod on Asa. He had to wake Asa up and completely change his pump site at 11pm. Once completed, he could then go recheck and give Aiden the insulin he needed. Dealing with one diabetic is hard. Dealing with more than one is more than unfair. Dealing with two who look identical to each other is mind-boggling!

Lessons Learned: Teach the twins the importance of staying in their own beds, and always lift the shirt to find the distinguishing mole.

Neither Diabetes nor children come with an instruction manual, and a lot is learned by trial-and-error. Diabetes is a frustrating continual balancing act, and sometimes one of the balls you are juggling gets dropped. Some days we feel like the protagonists in a comic strip, and Diabetes is the antagonist laughing at us. Sometimes I search for reasons for high or low sugars, and no plausible explanations exist.

Being a double-pancreas is not a job I signed up for. I was volun-told and dragged kicking and screaming into the role. Despite that, I take my job seriously, and "failures" like this are humbling and degrading. However, I try to stay positive and take away and learn from my own mistakes. We poke a little fun at each other, too, because if we do not laugh, we'll cry.

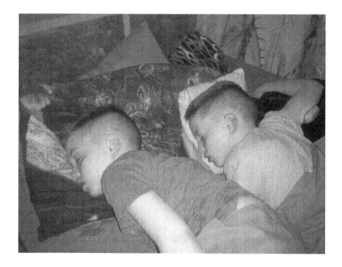

Who's Who?

Chapter Eleven: Tips and Advice

Learning to be a pancreas does not come with a manual. There is no one-size-fits-all way to manage this altered life, your home and this disease. However, I have found that doing a few things have helped make things easier on myself.

Get Organized

Once I wrapped my head around all this nonsense, getting organized was the only thing that made sense to me. First, I have one section in my kitchen where I store all the extra supplies. I have a plastic 4-drawer cart on the counter top that has all I need at any given time (Meters; Strips; Syringes; Alcohol; Flashlight; Glucose tabs; Batteries; Cotton balls; etc). In the cabinet above, I keep the educational materials and notebooks along with bulk overstock supplies (like boxes of alcohol and Omnipods).

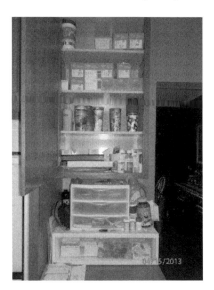

Diabetes Central

Second, I made a file on my computer for each boy. I have three forms. The first form has Basic Care Instructions that I can give to any caregiver in an emergency, or give to teachers each year (without having to recreate the wheel each time). Next, I have a Care Form that lists their current Insulin-to-Carb ratios, Basal rates (for the pumps), and Correction factors. Finally, I have an Overnight Care Form that I provide when the boys go stay the night somewhere. It has their current ratios, and a place for the caregiver to document glucose-carbs-insulin. (I updated all forms with any change, and the Overnight Care form is printed out each time the boys go visit Grandma or Sister).

Third, each boy has a binder and a clipboard that I use to file and store Diabetes-related care materials. Both are color-coded for each twin. Inside the notebook, I keep his completed weekly glucose logs, his Endocrinology reports, a nerdy flow chart tracking his A1Cs (aka Mommy Report Card), testing papers, and lab orders for the next Endocrinology visit. The clipboard is for the current week's blood glucose logs. Highs, lows and notes are highlighted in different colors on the clipboard so I can quickly identify a trend or pattern that needs to be investigated or tested.

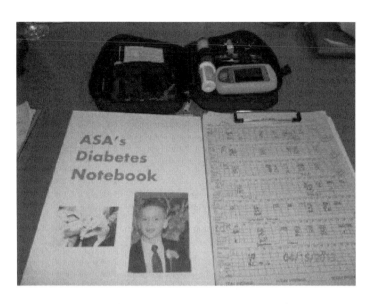

Example binder, clipboard and meter kit

Next, I have a Corkboard/Markerboard mounted in my kitchen. The Corkboard has the phone numbers to Pediatrician, CDEs and Endocrinology Clinic (so I don't have to look them up every time). It also has a list of basic supplies for D-bag (so I don't have to think – or forget—in a rushed situation). I post each boy's Care Form (so anyone, at a glance, can deliver the appropriate amounts of insulin for any given meal...and we are all on the same page)

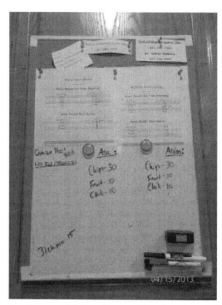

Corkboard/ Dry Erase Marker board combo

We use the Dry Erase Markerboard for keeping track of carbs at each meal. The Marker board has in permanent Sharpie the Pod Change Date (so we can remember, at a glance, when the next pod change is due), Asa and Aiden's name listed, so that carbs can be jotted down underneath their names at each meal, and "No Electronics for" line. This sweet little addition has really helped with managing behavior of all boys and keeping me on-track with consistent consequences because when my brain is swirling with insulin-carbs-glucose, I cannot always remember who lost privileges for how long!

Educate, Educate, Educate

As I've mentioned before, read everything you can get your hands on regarding Type One Diabetes. What they teach you in the hospital is only the basics. (They know your emotions are high, so they can only teach the basics - survival mode - because a newly diagnosed family would be overwhelmed with everything and unable to retain critical information). There is so much more to learn! Not everything will work for you or your child, but it helps tremendously to hear others' perspectives. The more you read about it, the more things begin to make sense. Take every class they offer. Attend seminars. Do whatever it takes to learn more.

Diabetes Education, like parenting, is a continuous process. The education you seek and receive should grow and change as the child grows and changes. Knowing how to manage Diabetes in a seven-year-old may vary widely from Diabetes management in a hormonal pubescent teenager. Further, the child with Diabetes needs to be involved in the educational process as much as possible. They need education that is age-appropriate and maturity-level appropriate. Currently, our boys listen to all discussion with the CDEs, read age-appropriate Diabetes books, and learn from what I explain to them. They are sharp. They get it, and they could probably teach many people a thing or two about Diabetes!

Open Communication with the School and other Caregivers

If your child goes to a public school, research and develop a 504 Plan. The term "504 Plan" refers to a plan developed to meet the requirements of a federal law that prohibits discrimination against people with disabilities, Section 504 of the Rehabilitation Act of 1973. There are many sample plans available online. It is used at any public or private school that receives government funding to assure a child is not discriminated against and is afforded the same opportunities for education as any child without an ailment. It is used at any public or private school that receives government funding. For us, our plan is pretty basic. It will be reviewed yearly with the school nurse, counselor and teachers to make sure we're all on the same page. All 504 plans should include assurance there are staff members trained to recognize hypoglycemia and hyperglycemia and to respond in accordance with the directions in the child's Diabetes Medical Management Plan (www.diabetes.org).

Visit with the school nurse and KNOW who is taking care of your child when he or she is at school. Let them know how you handle things, what you expect. I provide our school nurse with all supplies and snacks. We communicate daily. She sends me a report of how their days went and lets me know what supplies need to be refilled. I communicate back any changes we've made in their care or dosing.

Keep regular caregivers supplied with a kit that has strips, meters and low sugar supplies for an emergency. This also helps in case you forget or they run out while in their care. It is great if you keep a "Basics of Care" info sheet in that kit for reference.

Finally, participate in or encourage your child's teacher or nurse to educate the classmates about Type One Diabetes. If children understand, they tend to alienate less and ask less intrusive questions. Further, with a tiny bit of education, an astute student sitting next to your T1D child could alert the teacher of problems.

Be Prepared

Keep a Diabetes Bag packed and stocked. Our D-bag has a small provision of glucose tabs, a pouch of back-up supplies (strips, syringes, alcohol, and cotton), Carb Counting Book, Notepad & pen, and Glucagon. On any given trip, all we need to do is throw in their meter kits and we are good to go. We can add more snacks as needed depending on where we are going, what we are doing, and how long we will be gone. Furthermore, keep a list (like I do on the Corkboard) of what should always be in that bag so you do not overlook or forget something.

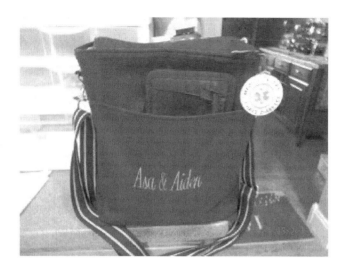

Keep hypoglycemia provisions in every nook and cranny you can think of. We keep glucose tabs, Smarties or a Quick Stick in every Diabetes-related bag (D-bag, meter kits, back packs), every vehicle glove compartment, and in my purse. As soon as you think you will sneak off for just a minute, that is when hypoglycemia will hit. You don't want to be caught with your pants down on this one! I have just "run to the store" with a boy who reports feeling low before we get to the end of the street! I give them the glucose source in my purse and when we return home and recheck, they are barely normal. Wow!

We have taught our boys that if they feel low on the school bus, use one of their snacks. We will deal with the glucose reading later. I am certain it has saved their lives more than once!

Halloween, Valentine's Day, Easter and Christmas are great times to **stock up** on individually packed candies that are perfectly portioned to treat low glucoses. Stock up at these times to keep these easy and tasty treats around for the times when hypoglycemia hits! They store well, travel well, and fit in their backpacks with ease. If your child has to have this crappy disease, at least he/she can treat hypoglycemia in a fun way!

Get Involved

Use your support system. Cry. Breathe. Align with people who understand and who are battling the same beast you are! It is great to get ideas and vent frustrations! I knew little about insulin pumps and nothing about CGMs and all the handy supplies we can use before I joined our Facebook forum!

Utilize your Endocrinology Clinic and Certified Diabetes Educators

Although they may not live the life, they do deal with Diabetes on a daily basis. They can help you think things through. This is routine for them, so they are accustomed to many questions, dumb questions and multiple questions. Do not be afraid to call. Do not be afraid to ask. It is their job!

If you or your child does not like your care team, find another one. You did not marry your Endocrinologist, but you can divorce from their care. You should neither expect nor accept judgment, condescension, or intimidation from any Diabetes care team member. Your child's Diabetes team should speak to them respectfully (since it's their disease) on a level they understand.

Getting organized, seeking education, open communication with all involved, and using all available resources can help you keep things straight and more effectively manage your child's Diabetes.

Conclusion

By all accounts, 2012 was a tough year for me, my family and my boys. Just when I thought I was reaching the Acceptance phase of grief after Aiden's diagnosis, Asa was diagnosed. The entire process started all over again. People may think it is not a big deal since you have traveled this road before, but frankly, I think it was even harder emotionally. I was in different phases of the same grieving process at the same time. Only a parent who has had their child diagnosed with this baffling disease can fully empathize with the emotional roller coaster it causes. Strap yourself in because it can be a bumpy ride. Diabetes is a strong foe, and it punches hard. I have always thought I was strong, and Diabetes has kicked me down yet made me stronger.

At the conclusion of my writing, we have now passed Aiden and Asa's one-year diaversaries. I have learned and accepted that Diabetes is a moving target, and hard as I try, I will never hit it! I have had to learn to be comfortable with a range of numbers instead of always wanting or expecting perfect numbers. I have tried so hard to make sense out of this illogical and nonsensical disease, and I have had to come to terms with the fact that I never will. As my husband said the other day, "Nothing surprises me anymore with this stupid disease." Our motto: Diabetes is stupid.

Diabetes has changed our lives. It is a part of their lives but does not define them. It is an ugly weed in the beautiful garden that is my boys' lives. However, with education, involvement, time and effort, I can keep those weeds at bay. Better treatments are being developed all the time, and a cure is on the horizon. I hope I live and my boys live to see the day when Elvis is forced to leave the building!

I have come to terms with and accepted that dealing with a child's illness is an extremely grueling process. Even after a year and a half, there are some days I am angry. Some days we sail. Some days I smile and feel victorious. Some days I cry. I cry when they pass milestones because they would not have lived to see the day in another time. I cry when I remember how much we all hurt upon Aiden's diagnosis. I cry when they get tired of it all because I cannot fix it. I cry with certain songs. I cry when I remember the feelings surrounding Asa's diagnosis. I cry when I am completely tired and exhausted. It is hard, but it gets easier.

Today, I am watching my boys grow and thrive by leaps and bounds. I am grateful they are alive and as healthy as can be. I am often puzzled and befuddled, but most days are good now. I do have my moments when the fatigue catches up to me, and I feel angry, confused, tearful and overwhelmed. I have to be strong for my boys.

The Acceptance phase of grieving has been reached, so we can focus on managing Diabetes as well as possible. Yet, the roller coaster ride will never end. It may get smoother, but it will not end until a cure is found. I know that now. So, in the words of Bon Jovi, "When the world gets in my face, I say 'Have a nice day'!"

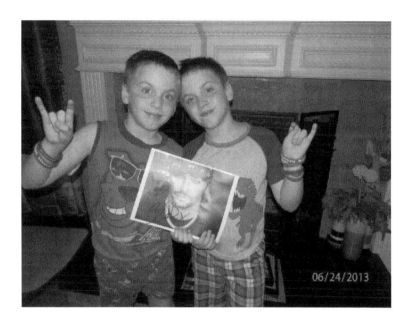

Asa and Aiden, inspired by an autographed picture of Bret Michaels (Type One Diabetic).

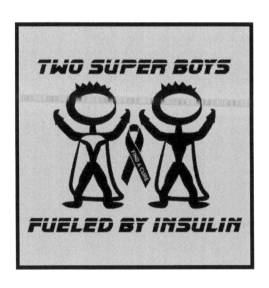

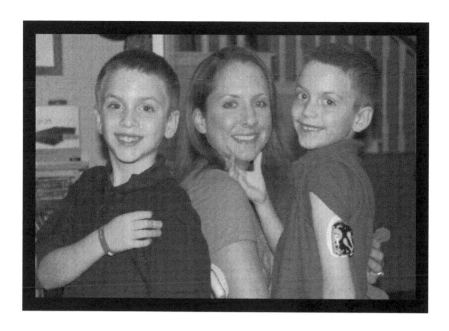

Asa and Aiden loved Mommy getting an Omnipod, too! We're in this together!

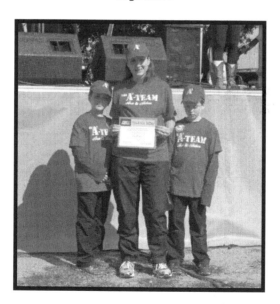

2013 The A2 Team for JDRF Walk to Cure Diabetes

Made in the USA
Lexington, KY
22 February 2015